How to understand and support children with

dyspraxia

Lois M. Addy

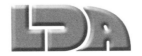

Acknowledgements

Many thanks to Dr Christine Mayers, Principal Lecturer, York St John College, University of Leeds, for her careful critique and constructive comments prior to the publication of this book.

Thank you to Glynnis Smith for her constructive advice regarding the Code of Practice.

Thank you to the children and adults who inspired the contents and who asked me to help others understand people with dyspraxia before trying to change them. In particular, thank you to Siobhan, Ben, Cherry, Katharine and Joe for their personal contributions.

Thank you to my family for their support; in particular Bethany and Charlotte who helped me to appreciate the pressures and joys of parenting, which has resulted in my being a more empathetic occupational therapist; and Geoff for his patience while I enthused about this subject.

How to understand and support children with dyspraxia
MT00603
ISBN-13: 978 1 85503 381 8
© Lois Addy
Cover illustration © Peter Wilks
Inside illustration © Janet Simmonett and Rebecca Barnes
All rights reserved
First published 2003
Reprinted 2004 (March, May, November), 2006, 2007

Printed in the UK for LDA
Abbeygate House, East Road, Cambridge, CB1 1DB, UK

Contents

Contents

Introduction

There is an increasing awareness amongst those working with children, be they teachers or therapists, of the rise in the number of children experiencing motor co-ordination and perceptual difficulties in primary and secondary education. Those difficulties have a profound effect on the child's ability to succeed within the structure of the National Curriculum.

Difficulties with co-ordination and perceptual processing have major repercussions on the child's handwriting legibility, organisation in the classroom and visual processing in relation to reading and numeracy, and in physical education. These limitations also have implications for self-image, which in turn is reflected in art and in personal appearance. Daily living skills such as dressing and feeding are also affected. Poor co-ordination of the muscles relating to speech can severely affect the child's expressive language, while comprehension is unaffected. Problems with oral control will also have an impact on eating and meal times can be a messy experience. Overall, this may have significant consequences for the child's peer relationships, social skills and self-confidence.

Children with dyspraxia have significant motor co-ordination and perceptual processing difficulties whilst retaining normal intelligence. Consequently they are acutely aware that the way they process, present and record information is different from that of their peers. This in turn results in low self-esteem and low self-confidence. The consequences of these processing problems are that many children with dyspraxia struggle with aspects of their educational experience and are hindered in achieving their potential. This has far-reaching effects on their adult life.

Dyspraxia is not a compelling handicap; it is not visible and it's hard to understand.
Dyspraxia Foundation

Dyspraxia is often termed the hidden handicap as there are no obvious signs of the child's dysfunction. They do not have any overt neurological signs as are evident in cerebral palsy, or a cluster of superficial features such as those seen with children with Down Syndrome. The child appears to be 'normal'.

It is when the children are asked to perform specific tasks that the extent of their visual perception and motor co-ordination difficulties becomes evident. Often, teachers initially observe that there seems to be a mismatch between the child's verbal reasoning and comprehension and their recorded work, the written work being extremely poor. They may also notice that the child is ungainly and uncoordinated in physical education and seems to be extremely clumsy in the classroom.

The author, in her capacity as a paediatric occupational therapist, has worked for twenty years with children with dyspraxia and has seen the extreme psychological effect that this condition can have on a child's self-esteem and self-confidence. It is hoped that by enabling readers to understand dyspraxia from the child's perspective, valuable insight can be gained which will encourage a collaborative approach to identifying solutions and strategies which can be implemented both in the classroom and at home.

The seemingly 'hidden' nature of dyspraxia and the extreme impact on a child's education are summarised in this poem by Katharine Jones, who captures how distressing dyspraxia was for her at school.

Dyspraxia is a pain

Dyspraxia is a pain!
It doesn't hurt.
I don't look different.
You can't see it . . .
Until breakfast.

I can't tie up my laces, and I always look
  a mess,
My shirt is buttoned wrongly –
I still find it hard to dress.
I can't hold my knife and fork yet,
I spill my drink, my mind is all muddled.
I know I am clumsy,
I get flustered and befuddled.

Dyspraxia is a pain!
It doesn't hurt.
I don't look different.
You can't see it . . .
Until I get into class.

I can't copy from the blackboard.
It's hard to concentrate.
The teachers call me lazy,
Keep me in and get irate.
They say that I'm untidy –
They're very quick to blame me and don't
  care to find out why.

Dyspraxia is a pain!
It doesn't hurt.
I don't look different.
You can't see it . . .
Until I write.

I can't write very neatly
And I can't write very small,
I get my letters backwards –
I can barely write at all.
The others say I'm stupid
And they call me lots of names,
They say that I'm a baby.
They won't let me share their games.

Dyspraxia is a pain!
It doesn't hurt.
I don't look different.

You can't see it . . .
Until it's art.

I can't cut out with scissors,
I can't rule nice straight lines.
I have never coloured neatly,
I don't draw good designs.
The other children mock me,
They think it's fun to tease –
They never want to play with me,
Like I've got some disease.

Dyspraxia is a pain!
It doesn't hurt.
I don't look different.
You can't see it . . .
Until I do PE.

I wobble when I balance,
It's awkward when I run.
I can't climb up a gym rope –
Sport isn't any fun.
I can't catch a bouncing football.
I can't kick one in the net.
I'm always 'it' when we play tag,
They jeer . . . I get upset.

Dyspraxia is a pain!
It doesn't hurt.
I don't look different.
But it really hurts inside.

I want to be like other children –
Good at sport and playing games.
I really want to score a goal.
I want to be the same;
I'd love to write so neatly
And be good at colouring in.
I want my work up on display
Not rejected in the bin.
I know that I am lucky;
I can walk and talk and play.
I just do it differently
And kids prefer the normal way.

*By kind permission of Katharine Jones,
aged 9*

In summary, this book will not:

- give the reader a remedy that will cure dyspraxia;
- recommend any specialist intervention over another;
- give the reader prescriptive strategies to meet the needs of children with dyspraxia.

The information contained in this book aspires to provide teachers, parents and health care professionals with the ability to:

- understand the needs of children with dyspraxia;
- understand why children with dyspraxia have difficulties in perceptual and motor planning;
- hear the problems of dyspraxia from a child's perspective;
- empathise with the frustrations of children with dyspraxia;
- demonstrate how classroom modifications can help;
- offer some solutions to specific problems faced by children with dyspraxia;
- recommend practical texts, programmes and equipment;
- supply some useful addresses and contacts.

Chapter 1
Common questions about dyspraxia

What is dyspraxia?

The term 'dyspraxia' is taken from the Greek *dys*, meaning ill, and *praxis*, meaning doing, acting, deed and practice – hence the literal meaning of 'dyspraxia' is ill-doing. This reflects the difficulties that children affected by it have in initiating and performing everyday tasks that many of us take for granted.

To understand this further, let us first consider the normal pattern of movement involved in a particular task.

Think of kicking a football, which on first thought appears easy. It involves a number of cognitive, perceptual and motor processes, all operating simultaneously. To carry out such a task successfully the individual first needs to understand the aim of the task, and then decide on the movements required. By consciously forming a mental image, a plan is formed which is then acted upon. The appropriate position is adopted, the balance is planned, the appropriate muscles are activated and the action is taken.

When a child learns to play with a football they must first grasp the idea of the movements required to kick it (ideation). This requires the child to visualise balancing on one leg whilst raising the other at the appropriate level and getting into a position close enough to the ball to strike it. To develop this mental image, previous experiences involving observed interactions with a ball and memory traces regarding similar personal experiences of ball play are brought to mind. Initial experiences demonstrated to the child are also recalled.

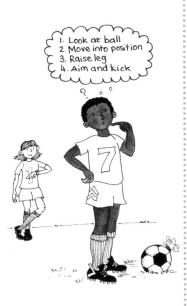

Secondly, the child needs to form a motor plan in order to place themselves in an appropriate position to kick the ball. They need to stand in front of the ball so they have a good view of the ball and the place they want to get it to. Appropriate balance is required prior to the movement. This involves co-ordination and organisation. It also requires prediction of the end result.

Thirdly, the child needs to carry out a sequence of movements to do the task. This involves raising one leg whilst the other retains balance, and extending the raised leg forwards with measured force to kick the ball to the desired place. This third stage is the execution of the task.

It is the mental imaging, planning and execution that enable functional skills to develop. In dyspraxia there is a problem in processing information which can occur at either one or all three stages.

Dyspraxia is, to sum up, impaired ability to conceptualise, organise and direct purposeful movement. It is not the motor skills *per se* that are influencing performance – as in, for example, cerebral palsy or muscular dystrophy (although many children with dyspraxia have low muscle tone or hypotonia). Rather it is impairment of conceptualising, planning and/or execution which is interfering with motor co-ordination.

It is therefore recommended that the term 'dyspraxia' should be used only in the following situations:

- When motor deficits are due to poor motor planning and organisation.
- When the motor deficits are significantly below the child's performance in other areas (Cermak, 1991).

Verbal dyspraxia is shown in a child who has difficulties in producing sounds, syllables and words. It is due to poor co-ordination of the oral structures – the lips, tongue and jaw. It is a difficulty in consciously organising the muscles required for speech rather than a muscular disorder.

Are there any other terms for dyspraxia?

A number of terms have been used to describe children who have marked motor co-ordination difficulties with additional problems in perceptual development and, occasionally, speech. These include:

- developmental agnosia and apraxia (Henderson and Hall, 1982);
- clumsy child syndrome (Gubbay, 1975);
- physically awkward, poorly co-ordinated (Cratty, 1994);
- perceptual–motor dysfunction (Laszlo *et al.*, 1988);
- sensory integrative dysfunction (Ayres, 1979);
- motor–learning disorder;
- deficit in attention, motor and perception (DAMP);
- minimal brain dysfunction;
- congenital maladroit;
- developmental apraxia;
- minimal cerebral palsy;
- minor neurological dysfunction;
- executive apraxia.

Developmental co-ordination disorder (DCD) is a relatively recent classification introduced to provide a recognisable diagnosis for those who have the following condition:

Marked impairment in the development of motor coordination that is not explainable by mental retardation and that is not due to a physical disorder. The diagnosis is only made if this impairment significantly interferes with academic achievement or with activities of daily living (APA,1994).

DCD is an umbrella term covering several presentations. Dyspraxia is a type of developmental co-ordination disorder.

Dyspraxia is the term perhaps used more commonly by teachers, parents and health care professionals. In 1985 the Dyspraxia Foundation described dyspraxia as follows:

> An impairment or immaturity in the organisation of planned movement with associated problems of perception, and occasionally speech.

This introduces speech disorder, which is defined as follows:

> Developmental verbal dyspraxia (DVD) is an articulation disorder that can affect speech sound production and non-speech movements. Children with DVD have difficulty in planning, initiating and executing speech sounds and non-speech movements. It is a motor programming problem, not a muscular weakness (Hill, 2003).

The term 'dyspraxia' throughout this book refers to a difficulty in planning and carrying out motor acts. It emphasises that the problem is one of motor and perceptual organisation, difficulties in which can significantly affect the child's ability in the classroom.

How many children with dyspraxia will there be in my class?

Research has shown that 5.3 per cent of the population suffer from problems of co-ordination and do not achieve their academic potential (Maeland, 1992; Gubbay, 1975; Henderson and Hall, 1982). Others consider the figure is as high as 10 per cent (Laszlo and Bairstow, 1985; Cratty, 1979). From these findings, it can be assumed that at least 1 child in a class of 30 will have motor co-ordination difficulties, but the figure may rise to as many as 3.

Are children with dyspraxia mostly boys?

Dyspraxia affects more boys than girls. Figures indicate that boys are four times more likely than girls to be referred for assessment, therapy and specialist teaching (Henderson, 1993; Portwood, 1999). It is not known why this is the case. Gillberg (1995) suggests it is to do with different developmental patterns for males and females.

Other studies have demonstrated that girls tend to be more precise in their fine motor activities while boys are faster but less accurate (Grant and Watter, 1998). These characteristics are often seen in pre-school children, with boys preferring gross motor play. In a child with dyspraxia, it is likely that these differences are exaggerated.

What causes dyspraxia?

The causes of dyspraxia are unclear, but it is fundamentally a neurodevelopmental disorder resulting from an immaturity in the developing brain. There are a number of reasons why this might occur:

- A lack of oxygen around the time of birth, an early viral infection, or alcohol or poison abuse such as foetal alcohol syndrome (Lee and French, 1994).

- There is evidence that premature birth leads to the failure of the neurones in the brain to form adequate connections. This has an effect on the brain's ability to process information (Brooks-Gunn *et al.*, 1992; Padsman *et al.*, 1998).

- Dyspraxia can result from an inability to bring together sensory information. This affects the ability to develop body schemas for motor planning.

- Some studies have found a genetic or familial link, but no evidence has been found to indicate chromosomal abnormalities (Johnstone *et al.*, 1987).

How can I recognise a child with dyspraxia?

Not all of the characteristics shown here will be found in every child with dyspraxia; each child will have their own individual profile. However, at various ages a number of signs may be identified. These are displayed in the lists supplied.

Pre-school

The following characteristics are typical:

- Delay in acquiring normal motor milestones, for example delayed walking.

- Children with dyspraxia have difficulties in balance and may be unable to hop, skip or maintain continuous movements in order to jump well. This in turn affects their ability to play ball games.

- Poor spatial organisation; a child with dyspraxia will tend to bump into objects because of their inability to judge distances accurately.

- Difficulties in constructive play; for example manipulating Lego® bricks.

- Untidy appearance due to poor body image and an inability to co-ordinate dressing and undressing.

- Inability to manage a knife and fork, resorting to fingers whenever possible.

- If the child has verbal dyspraxia, they will have produced little or no babbling in infancy.

- The pre-school child may show poor expressive language despite having good verbal comprehension.

- Children with dyspraxia are often heavy handed and heavy footed and may resort to walking on tiptoe when moving at speed. This may be due to low muscle tone.

- Lack of rhythm in movement.

❍ Sensitivity to noisy environments.

❍ Delayed toilet training.

Key Stages 1 and 2

Characteristics are as follows:

❍ Difficulty in fastening their clothes, for example doing up buttons and tying shoe laces. They have difficulty getting ready for physical education on time.

❍ General organisation may be erratic.

❍ Inability to undertake activities without seeing their hands, for example combing hair, wiping bottom.

❍ Frequently bump into things.

❍ Difficulty in physical education relating to hopping, jumping and balancing, ball skills and swimming.

❍ Trip over easily.

❍ Dislike playing in playgrounds or on apparatus.

❍ Difficulty performing bilateral activities such as sewing, using scissors, using a knife and fork.

❍ Poor self-awareness.

❍ Confusion between left and right.

❍ Poor drawing and constructional skills.

❍ Erratic handwriting with many reversals and poorly formed letters.

❍ Reading may appear to deteriorate as the child grows older.

❍ Poor spacing of words on a page.

❍ Difficulty with numeracy.

❍ Poor written content despite evidence of knowledge through discussion.

❍ Low self-esteem.

❍ Frustration when several things happen at once.

❍ Often distractible, with a tendency to daydream.

❍ May have a short attention span or difficulty in concentrating.

❍ May be a loner or disruptive in class.

❍ Difficulty in copying text from a book or the board.

❍ Children with verbal dyspraxia will have difficulties with expressive language.

❍ Reading development may be affected in children with verbal dyspraxia. The child may know which letters to say but cannot sequence them to form words.

- Intonation in children with verbal dyspraxia may be unusual and speech may sound fragmented and sluggish.

- Social skills may be poor and the child may make friendships with children younger than themselves.

- The child is more vulnerable to bullying and being manipulated by other children.

- Eating habits can be poor, which may affect peer acceptance.

Key Stages 3 and 4

The following characteristics may be seen:

- Inability to write quickly and maintain the pace of their peers.

- Reading appears to become more difficult. This tends to be due to the size of the print, the volume of print on the page and occasionally the starkness in contrast between the white page and black print.

- Disorganisation may be evident, especially as the child is trying to understand the various dimensions of a complex timetable, more subjects, a larger establishment and a variety of room locations.

- Children with dyspraxia may have difficulty in taking dictation or recalling detailed instructions.

- Physical education in Key Stages 3 and 4 tends to incorporate more team games, which may prove problematic due to the spatial organisation required and the competitive nature of these games.

- Design technology with its conceptualisation of three dimensions may be affected by poor spatial organisation.

- Difficulties in taking notes from the board.

- Laboured handwriting may result in children taking their work home with them to finish, a problem which is exacerbated by the increasing requirement for creative written material in the secondary school setting.

- Children with dyspraxia often have low self-esteem, which will affect their academic achievement.

- Continued poor speech production in children with verbal dyspraxia. This is likely to have an impact on the child's relationships and self-confidence.

Can dyspraxia be cured?

There is no cure for dyspraxia, but children can certainly be helped to learn new skills, refine the skills already acquired or compensate for their difficulties.

Do children grow out of dyspraxia?

In general, children do not 'grow out' of dyspraxia, as was previously thought. Children can and do learn to accommodate their difficulties and there is clear evidence that early intervention can have beneficial results (Losse *et al.*, 1991).

*Low self-esteem is
like driving through
life with your
handbrake on.*
Maxwell Maltz

Children who do not receive help suffer from low self-esteem and low self-confidence and this will have far-reaching effects on their academic potential.

Can anything be done to help?

The good news is that there are a variety of approaches and techniques which can be used to help children with dyspraxia to overcome their difficulties. Some aspects of their development can be learned, certain aspects changed and others accommodated by using adaptations or compensatory strategies.

It is important that each child's needs are considered individually. It is also preferable that the child is helped at a young age. Perceptual responsiveness is best addressed between the ages of 4 and 8 years. The research that underpinned the *Write from the Start* programme (Addy, 1995) demonstrated that children's perceptual development in relation to handwriting can be radically altered if the child's needs are addressed in their early school years.

For teachers and others who work with children with dyspraxia, an understanding of how the children perceive their world is essential. How each child interprets their environment is fundamental to turning the key to unlock their potential. Therefore educating the professionals and carers is an essential component of assisting these children.

More details will be given in later chapters of this book regarding the various approaches which can be adopted.

To begin with, we look at the development of motor co-ordination and perception and see how it can go wrong, causing many of the difficulties children with dyspraxia face.

Chapter 2
The development of motor skills and perception

I am slatternly; I seldom put and never keep things in order; I am careless; I forget rules; I read when I should learn my lessons; I have no method and sometimes . . . I cannot bear to be subjected to systematic arrangements. Said by Helen Burns in Charlotte Bronte's *Jane Eyre*

Children with dyspraxia are typically recognised by their lack of motor co-ordination. They are often heavy footed and seem to bump into everything. They are physically awkward and are reluctant to take part in activities in physical education lessons.

In order to address the needs of these children it is important to understand why they have these difficulties. Often a simple appreciation of how and what the children perceive can give insight into the confusion and frustration they feel.

The development of motor co-ordination

Early stages of development

When a new baby enters the world their movements appear uncoordinated. They are very much influenced by the continued presence of primitive reflexes. Many of these reflexes can be felt by the mother when the baby is still in the womb. She experiences these through kicks, squirming and rolls. These movements serve an important purpose in that they help young children develop an awareness of their bodies whilst experiencing stretching (extending) and bending (flexing) of their limbs. Several of these reflexes have a part to play during birth and beyond as the baby begins to develop.

Many of these reflexes disappear immediately after birth but some persist for several months as they help in survival. An example is the rooting reflex, which can be seen by softly touching the sides of the child's mouth. This prompt causes the child to turn towards the stimulus and in the event of the nipple touching leads them to their mother's milk.

Certain reflexes such as the Moro reflex help to develop body schema and symmetry. In the Moro reflex, the baby spreads the arms and legs wide and extends the neck in response to a noise or quick change in position. Early motor responses rely on the presence of such reflexes.

Primitive reflexes are replaced by more advanced equilibrium, righting and saving reactions. These enable children to begin to move against gravity, and to develop a symmetrical posture.

Take the child who is beginning to sit. If pushed forwards or sideways they will extend their arm to save themselves from falling. This allows them to maintain an upright posture in order to use their arms, legs and head for purposeful movement.

The ability to support the body and to prop yourself on extended arms is very important. It enhances another motor function essential for refined motor development, that of proprioception.

Proprioception

Proprioception is the awareness of where our limbs are in space. Within our muscles and joints we have sensitive receptors which react to the amount of contraction or stretch our muscles undergo when moving. These receptors inform our brain how much the muscle is responding and this is recorded for future use in our memory system.

For example, when a baby reaches for a rattle, the amount of stretch the child has to undertake in order to grasp the rattle is relayed and recorded in the brain's motor memory. Therefore when a toy is seen again in the same position, the child is able to reach out to grasp the toy, using the information gained about the amount of muscle stretch and contraction necessary. Receptors are located all over our body, giving us a constant map in our minds of our whole body's position. This is vital information for controlled movement to take place.

As this system develops, children eventually become aware of where their limbs are without needing to look at them. This is essential for many functional tasks such as brushing the back of our hair, cleaning after toileting and tucking in the back of a shirt.

We know that in children with dyspraxia the neurones of the brain fail to form adequate connections, which results in processing difficulties. This is apparent when considering proprioception; the majority of children with dyspraxia have poor proprioception. The reason for this is not fully known, but what tends to happen is that the information regarding muscle stretch and relaxation becomes less clear, causing the child to have an inaccurate perception of where their limbs are in space. This has a strong influence on motor control as it makes accurate placement of the feet, hands and trunk difficult. The movements appear heavy and the child begins to appear clumsy.

In addition, children with dyspraxia may not be fully aware of exactly where their arms and legs are in relation to their trunk without looking at them. As a consequence tasks where they cannot see their limbs are rarely achieved well. Dressing can appear messy and hair unkempt, and toilet hygiene may be poor.

This inability to control muscle position can affect the application of pressure through the limbs; often children with dyspraxia will either press too hard or not hard enough when writing or undertaking a construction task.

Vestibular system

Our vestibular apparatus provides us with information regarding the direction and speed of movement.

The inner ear contains the complex structures of the semi-circular canals, the vestibule and cochlea being two of these. These form the core of the vestibular apparatus. Tiny hairs located within our ear wave to and fro according to the movement of our head. Electrochemical impulses from these hairs send messages along nerve pathways to our brain, which interprets direction of movement and speed. Even while we are standing in an upright position, these hairs wave slightly.

The importance of this system will be evident if you have ever suffered an inner-ear infection. The symptoms experienced include loss of balance, a feeling of nausea and insecurity on our feet. In this situation it is preferable to sit down or reduce movement as far as possible.

The function of this system is to detect the speed and direction of our body's movement. It enables us to maintain an upright position, maintain muscle tone, and adjust ourselves according to position and movement without losing our balance.

Many children with dyspraxia receive messages through the vestibular system that don't make sense. This leaves them uncoordinated, lacking control of the speed of their movements. This can be seen in physical education when children are asked to run around the room and then stop on command. Children with dyspraxia will often overrun through lack of vestibular control, in what appears to be an overflow of movement.

Having vestibular and proprioceptive systems that do not function as they should can lead to children appearing very clumsy and uncoordinated. It may account for why children with dyspraxia experience difficulties with fine motor control and the adjustment of pressure through the hands and feet. It may also explain their preference to sit down rather than stand upright.

Sensory system

The sensory system provides another way of getting detailed information about our environment and how to respond to it. Communication to the central nervous system begins when input from the environment stimulates the sensory receptors.

There are many receptors which are responsible for relaying this input, providing us with evidence about our surroundings. All of this information is taken to the cortex of the brain where the receptors have their own unique receiver. The incoming information will enable us to detect temperature, pressure, light, size, texture, sound and so on.

In children with dyspraxia, there are difficulties in relation to these senses. The connections in the brain do not work properly and cause the response to the information to become dampened down or too great. This will add to the confusion the child feels in their environment and may account for much unusual behaviour as the child tries to cope with their experiences.

In relation to touch, for example, the child may be very sensitive and clothes may feel itchy. Close contact with others in the lunch queue may feel uncomfortable.

Alternatively, they may have low sensitivity to touch and crave physical contact in order to stabilise their own position and sense of where they are in space. These children are likely to crash around and bump into things frequently. Grips on objects may be extreme; when writing the pencil grip may be tight and pressure through the pencil heavy. They may be found constantly fiddling with objects or chewing.

The development of perception

Children with dyspraxia will experience perceptual difficulties as a result of their motor co-ordination, proprioception and sensory integration difficulties. However, each child will show a range of difficulties, some greater than others.

Each child is an individual and will have their own profile; therefore it must not be assumed that all of the following aspects of perception will be delayed or dysfunctional.

Hand–eye co-ordination

Hand–eye co-ordination, or visual–motor co-ordination as it is often termed, is the ability to co-ordinate a hand movement to a visual goal. Whenever we reach for an object our vision guides our hand to the goal. This is one of the earliest levels of perceptual development, acquired during early infancy.

As hand–eye co-ordination develops, other areas of perception, such as spatial organisation and motor planning, are required. With their help, objects can be picked up carefully and put down in a precise position.

Problems with hand–eye co-ordination occur when proprioception and vestibular feedback are not as accurate as they should be. The systems provide incorrect information about the location of the arm and hand, and about the degree of movement required to reach an object. As a consequence, the development of precise motor control is restricted.

Children who have problems in this area will find even the simplest tasks difficult to perform. They will find dressing and undressing difficult owing to the complexity of managing fastenings. Placement of blocks on top of one another or of pegs in a board will also prove problematic. Tasks such as handwriting, cooking and baking, and even the use of a knife and fork, may be difficult.

Children experiencing such difficulties often feel inadequate because of their failure to achieve even the simplest activities for daily living. This may result in low self-esteem and possibly avoidance of certain tasks.

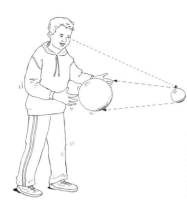

Figure 1. Perception of a child whose visual constancy is established.

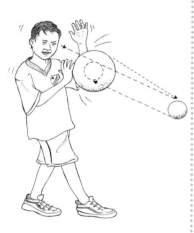

Figure 2. Perception of a child whose visual constancy is distorted.

Form constancy

A person with adequate form constancy will recognise a cube even when it is viewed from an oblique angle. Likewise a table viewed from a number of angles will still be recognised as a table.

This area of perceptual development follows that of hand–eye co-ordination and occurs at about 5 months. During this period an understanding of shape variations is beginning to form, and as a baby holds an object and twists and turns it, the discovery is made that the object is solid.

The ability to recognise an object or form when it is presented in a different size is also part of form constancy. For example, when copying from the board children need to understand that the letter shape written on the board is the same form as that written in their books. In a similar way, when playing football, children must be able to recognise that the football viewed several metres away, despite seeming smaller, is the same ball as that which was kicked moments earlier.

As children with dyspraxia are often receiving the wrong information regarding touch, weight, texture and visual dimension, recognition of form can prove problematic so that categories of shape, form and size are not easily identified.

Dysfunction in this area of perception can result in major difficulties, with children unable to order the sizes and forms they view. Their environment will appear extremely unstable. A similar object may appear completely different if altered even slightly. This can often be seen in writing tasks, where letter shapes appear to be formed erratically. It can be seen more significantly when a child with dyspraxia attempts ball skills. The ball that they recognise as a certain size in one location may appear totally different when at a distance. Consequently when a ball is thrown to them they are unable to adjust to the actual size of the ball (see Figs. 1 and 2).

Visual figure–ground discrimination

Figure–ground discrimination is the ability to select and focus on one item or object despite the mass of visual stimuli that is around us. The 'figure' is the part of the visual field that holds our attention. When the attention is shifted onto something different, the previous figure recedes into the background.

An object or figure cannot be perceived unless it is seen in relation to a background. Therefore, a child playing with a group of friends in a park could not perceive another child and their position unless they are viewed against background objects such as the swings, slide, roundabout and ground.

Distorted figure–ground perception has a severe effect on reading, attention and organisation. This is because the visual stimuli (and auditory stimuli) can simply appear overwhelming. The attention is drawn to every stimulus and focusing on just one, excluding the background stimuli, becomes very difficult.

Children with poor figure–ground perception will be attracted to any interesting object – something that moves, something glittery, something brightly coloured. In short, their world is a mass of interesting objects, each as important as the others.

For a child with dyspraxia, this affects the ability to read. Initially reading develops well, but as the letter font decreases and words per page increase, it becomes more difficult for them to follow the text. All the words come forward into focus. Children with these difficulties will also have problems sorting objects, identifying items within a cluttered or busy work or home situation and attending within a large group, especially if the environment is noisy. They will have difficulty in following some workbooks – especially those used in numeracy, which can appear cluttered.

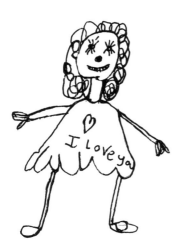

Figure 3. 'Me' by Bethany, aged 5 years.

Position in space

Position in space is a further aspect of perception which develops as proprioception and vision become refined. It is the ability to perceive or view oneself in relation to another object or person. It incorporates the understanding of spatial concepts such as *above, below* and *beneath* and the appreciation of where things are placed in relation to a central figure.

Most children with dyspraxia have a poor sense of position in space, yet their understanding of spatial concepts is good. With many children with dyspraxia these concepts cannot be described but can be located.

For example, if a child is asked to 'put the spoon under the box', they may be able to do this easily. If asked, 'Where is the spoon?' they may be unable to choose the correct term to describe the concept of 'under'.

In order to relate ourselves to another object an accurate body schema is required. This is a sense of where your body is in space, for example where the arms are in relation to the trunk. A sense of body schema develops through the response of muscles, proprioception and tactile experiences, along with other sensations. All these provide a map or picture of how we think we look.

It is through this information that we can perceive ourselves as symmetrical and appropriately proportioned. We can also understand laterality in that we have a left and right side which can work together or independently. An intact body schema can be assessed by asking someone to draw a picture of themselves. Although young children may lack certain features and details, an intact body schema and perception of position in space can be seen in their drawings. The drawing by Bethany (Fig. 3) shows that she has a good sense of position in space.

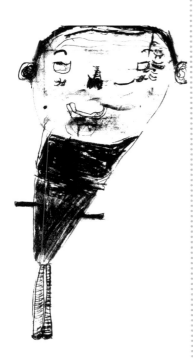

Figure 4. Self-portrait by Helen, aged 10 years.

Distorted perception of position in space will result in the child having a distorted or primitive body awareness, as can be seen in the drawing by Helen (Fig. 4). She is unable to see the shapes and patterns that come together to form her eyes and nose; instead she fragments each part. Proportion is often erratic, and body parts are often missed out.

Children with these difficulties will often lack an awareness of their appearance. Shirts will often be untucked, tidiness will be compromised, and children with body schemas similar to Helen's will find it very difficult to tidy their hair. Clothes that are put on inside out or back to front and shoes that are put on the wrong feet also show distorted perception in this area.

In addition to affecting their appearance, an inability to distinguish symmetry will affect the child's idea of laterality. They will have difficulty in knowing left and right. This will be reflected in orientation and will affect letter writing, resulting in frequent letter reversals. Mirror writing may occur and reversed letters may appear within words. The children may start writing from the right side of the page, proceeding to the left.

Spatial relationships

This involves the ability to perceive the position of two or more objects in relation to ourselves and in relation to each other.

For example, when playing football in the position of goalkeeper, the whole field can be scanned and a picture made up of exactly where all the players are situated, how far they are from each other and how far they are from the goal (Fig. 5). In this way, preparation can be made to move swiftly into the most appropriate position.

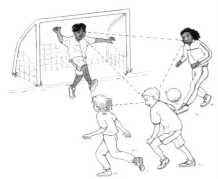

Figure 5. Spatial judgement required while playing football.

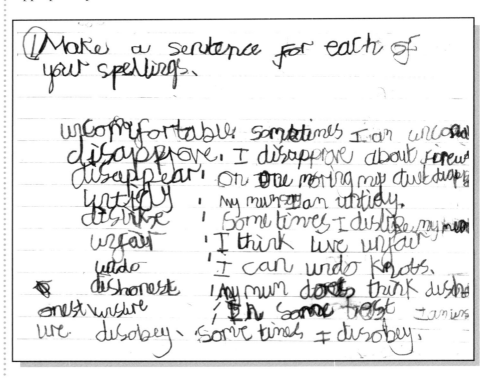

Figure 6. Example of writing demonstrating spatial organisation difficulties.

Difficulties in spatial organisation are commonly seen in children with dyspraxia. This is why they seem to bump into things frequently, and appear clumsy.

Difficulties in this area of visual perception will also have an effect on writing ability. Children may omit spaces between words; they may commence writing in the centre of the page or write in a diagonal direction rather than horizontal (Fig. 6). Overall this will result in illegibility and can lead to frustration on the part of the teacher who is attempting to read the work. Mathematics may prove problematic as the presentation and layout of calculations can easily be misplaced, affecting the end result (Fig. 7).

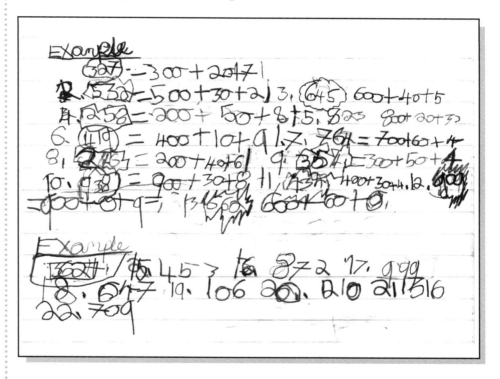

Figure 7. Example of calculations demonstrating spatial organisation difficulties.

Visual closure

Visual closure is a form of perception whereby an object can be identified even though its outline has been fragmented. The parts come together to enable the whole to be seen.

It is because of this perceptual dimension that letters can be seen individually within a word, but also that the word can be seen as a whole.

Children with difficulties in visual closure will have problems with handwriting activities, construction tasks and general classroom organisation. When writing, they will tend to focus on the individual components of the letter rather than the letter as a whole unit; for example, the letter *a* may be written as 'O I'. Their problems will make jigsaw puzzles difficult due to an inability to see the connection between parts of a picture. Items partly hidden within a room may be impossible to find.

The combined aspects of hand–eye co-ordination, form constancy, visual figure–ground discrimination, position in space, spatial relationships and visual closure enable us to make sense of the world around us and develop self-awareness and control.

Many of the areas of perception outlined overlap with one another and it may be hard to decide which aspect is stopping the child from successfully completing certain tasks. However, through observing the child perform simple activities it becomes possible to determine where the specific problem lies. A number of observation tasks and simple activities are included in the next chapter to help identify the child's difficulties in relation to perception.

This chapter has outlined the effect that motor and perceptual difficulties can have on children with dyspraxia. What is harder to convey is how the child is feeling as a result of such difficulties and the effect such problems can have on the child's self-esteem and confidence. This is revealed in the following poem.

My life

I get up in the morning,
My head's in a spin.
I don't want to get up,
Don't want the day to begin.

I have my breakfast,
I make a mess.
I have a wash,
Then it's time to dress.

It takes me ages to get myself dressed.
My clothes go on wrong
Though I try my best.

My mum takes me to school.
I go off to my class,
I struggle through my work —
I wish the time would pass.

My writing is messy,
My drawings are too.
I don't like my paintings,
I wish I was like you.

I go outside at playtime,
No one will play with me
Because I can't run fast enough.
I wish I was watching TV.

I wish my life wasn't this hard,
I wish it was more fun.
I wish nobody laughed at me —
I'd like a friend, just one.

I'd like to play more sports
But I'm never picked for teams.
I wish I could be better
Like I am in my dreams.

Tomorrow might be a nicer day,
I hope I make a friend.
I'd like to be more lucky,
I wish unhappiness would end.

By kind permission of Ben Cooper, aged 10

Chapter 3
Assessment and identification

When is dyspraxia likely to be recognised?

The child with dyspraxia usually comes to the attention of professionals at the age of 4 or 5 when they begin full-time education. Very quickly the teacher begins to see that the child's motor co-ordination is somewhat lacking and that their verbal skills are far more advanced than their manual abilities.

The role of the SENCo

The teacher will, no doubt, seek advice from the school's special educational needs co-ordinator (SENCo), who will consider the needs of the child in consultation with the teacher and parents. The SENCo is invaluable in offering advice about how the child's difficulties can be addressed in school. If further advice is required, the SENCo may discuss the child's progress with other professionals and may refer them to the local Child Development Centre. Alternatively, parents may be advised to go through their general practitioner to gain such a referral.

If the child is referred to the local Child Development Centre, a more detailed assessment will be carried out, often using standardised assessments. These will include assessment of the child's perceptual, cognitive and motor skills, along with a review of the child's abilities in daily living skills as well as their emotional well-being.

What to look out for

At the initial stages, information should be collected regarding the child's motor skills, reading ability and manual dexterity. The informal approach of observation is a good idea; an initial checklist is included on page 24. Once more information is known, the teacher will have a better understanding of the child's needs and will be in a good position to address these needs using the suggestions provided in the following chapters.

Informal assessment

Initially assessment can be undertaken through observation, the teacher or parent answering the questions supplied.

If answers to questions 1 to 16 are mostly 'Yes' and answers to questions 17 to 26 mostly 'No', it is likely that the child has some degree of dyspraxia.

For more specific assessments in the areas of handwriting, numeracy, physical education, reading and social skills the checklists on pages 25–29 may prove useful to identify specific areas of difficulty. An observation list for verbal dyspraxia is also offered (page 30).

Initial checklist

	Observation	Yes	No
1.	Does the child have difficulty holding a pencil?		
2.	Does the child have difficulty forming letters?		
3.	Are the child's drawings distorted or immature?		
4.	Does the child appear clumsy?		
5.	Is the child easily distracted?		
6.	Does the child appear unaware of their appearance and look unkempt?		
7.	Does the child have poor attention skills?		
8.	Does the child have difficulty getting organised?		
9.	Does the child have difficulty manoeuvring around objects?		
10.	Does the child often seem confused or frustrated?		
11.	Does the child seem to have low self-esteem or little self-confidence?		
12.	Does there appear to be a mismatch between the child's verbal reasoning and written recording?		
13.	Are the child's letter sizes erratic?		
14.	Does the child have difficulty in communicating?		
15.	Does the child's speech deteriorate under pressure; for example when put on the spot for an answer?		
16.	Does the child have poor oral control when eating?		
17.	Can the child hop?		
18.	Can the child jump with two feet together?		
19.	Is the child able to balance on one leg?		
20.	Can the child thread beads?		
21.	Can the child cut with scissors?		
22.	Can the child use a ruler effectively?		
23.	Can the child dress and undress for physical education?		
24.	Can the child manoeuvre on and off physical education apparatus?		
25.	Does the child leave adequate spaces between words when writing a sentence?		
26.	Does the child commence writing at the appropriate side of the page?		

Handwriting checklist

	Observation	Yes	No
1.	Does the child seem unsure which hand to hold the pencil in?		
2.	Is the pencil held in an abnormal grip?		
3.	Does the child sit appropriately on a chair when writing?		
4.	Does the child slump forward onto the table when writing?		
5.	Does the child position the paper awkwardly when writing?		
6.	Does the child lift their wrist off the paper when writing?		
7.	Is too much pressure applied through the pencil?		
8.	Is too little pressure applied through the pencil?		
9.	Are letters formed appropriately?		
10.	Are reversed or inverted letters evident?		
11.	Does the child commence writing at the left side of the page?		
12.	Does the writing slope downwards across a page rather than follow a horizontal direction?		
13.	Are inadequate spaces left between words?		
14.	Are the sizes of letters erratic?		
15.	Are letters incompletely formed, i.e. the cross bar is missing from the 't'?		
16.	Does the child's writing contain an erratic mixture of upper- and lower-case lettering?		
17.	Do you struggle to identify distinct ascenders and descenders in the child's writing?		
18.	Does the child struggle to join letters appropriately?		
19.	Does writing appear slow and laboured?		
20.	Is the speed of writing slow?		
21.	Does the child have low writing confidence?		

Numeracy checklist

	Observation	Yes	No
1.	Does the child understand spatial concepts such as top, bottom, above, below, inside, beside?		
2.	Is the child able to recite numbers in the correct order?		
3.	Is the child able to write numbers in the correct sequence?		
4.	Can the child write numbers in the correct orientation?		
5.	Does the child seem confused when there is more than one problem on a page or when the page has additional information such as pictures and patterns on it?		
6.	Does the child struggle to set out calculations correctly?		
7.	Is the child able to calculate age-appropriate sums mentally?		
8.	Is the child confused by the meaning of certain mathematical symbols?		
9.	Is the child confused by mathematical terms which mean the same thing – for example times and multiply?		
10.	Does the child rely on fingers or objects to count?		
11.	Does the child struggle to count objects due to poor organisation?		
12.	Can the child match three-dimensional objects to a corresponding picture?		
13.	Does the child struggle to depict three-dimensional objects?		
14.	Does the child understand the direction of calculations? For example when adding 100s, 10s and units presented in columns, do they remember to start from the right?		
15.	Is the child able to estimate or suggest an approximate figure when looking at a series of objects?		
16.	Can the child manipulate practical maths equipment effectively – for example Cuisenaire® rods?		
17.	Can the child control a ruler in order to draw shapes or straight lines?		
18.	Can the child remember simple number rules when taught in the class?		

Physical education checklist

	Observation	Yes	No
1.	Does the child race around large spaces such as a gym hall in an uncontrolled manner?		
2.	Does the child appear intimidated by the space and sounds of a large hall and prefer to stay on the edges?		
3.	Does the child bump into other group members whenever an activity requiring movement is undertaken?		
4.	When controlled movement is required, does the child demonstrate an overflow of movement; for example when running around the hall, if 'stop' is called, will the child run on?		
5.	Is the child able to hop?		
6.	Is the child able to jump on the spot with two feet together?		
7.	Is the child able to jump forward?		
8.	Is the child able to skip?		
9.	When throwing an object such as a ball or beanbag, is there a lack of control and direction?		
10.	Is the child able to catch a ball?		
11.	Is the child able to balance on all four limbs?		
12.	Is the child able to balance on all four limbs and raise an arm and opposite leg from the floor without falling over?		
13.	Is the child able to balance on all four limbs and raise an arm and leg from the same side of the body without falling over?		
14.	Is the child able to balance on one knee without toppling over?		
15.	Is the child reluctant to use apparatus which takes them off the floor; for example walking along a gym bench or climbing over a horse?		
16.	Does running appear clumsy and uncoordinated?		
17.	Is the child reluctant to join in team games?		
18.	Is co-ordination when moving around objects poor?		
19.	Does the child prefer activities based at floor level?		

Reading checklist

	Observation	Yes	No
1.	Has the child's reading seemed to deteriorate over their time in school?		
2.	Does the child become tired when reading?		
3.	Does the child rub their eyes frequently when reading?		
4.	Does the child lose their place on the page easily?		
5.	Does the child tend to repeat words previously read due to an inability to scan along each row?		
6.	Does the child skip rows when reading?		
7.	Does the child struggle to read information when the font is small?		
8.	Does the child struggle to read when the page appears to have a considerable amount of information on it?		
9.	Does the child struggle to sound out words?		
10.	Does reading improve if the print is in a colour other than black?		
11.	Does reading improve if words are written on a coloured background?		
12.	Does the child ever complain of headaches or nausea when reading?		
13.	Does the child struggle to concentrate to read for more than a few minutes?		
14.	Does the child use excessive head movement when reading?		
15.	Does the child hold their head at an angle when reading?		
16.	Does the child lie across the table on one arm when reading?		
17.	Does the child try to avoid reading?		

Social skills & communication checklist

	Observation	Yes	No
1.	Is there a difficulty for the child in initiating conversation?		
2.	Does the child show difficulty in adapting to new or unfamiliar situations?		
3.	In unpredictable situations, will the child react by – for example – bursting into tears or lashing out?		
4.	In group situations is the child placid or overcontrolling?		
5.	Are there problems with personal hygiene (often due to poor toilet hygiene)?		
6.	Does the child show difficulty in picking up non-verbal signs, which may lead to tactless statements being made?		
7.	Does the child show difficulty with listening skills owing to being distracted?		
8.	Is there a tendency for the child to opt out when things appear too difficult?		
9.	Is the child sensitive to failure?		
10.	Does the child have a difficulty in understanding certain types of humour, particularly sarcasm?		
11.	Does the child have emotional outbursts during periods of great stress?		
12.	Does the child have difficulty in appreciating the viewpoint of others?		
13.	Does the child struggle to find a range of solutions to problems?		
14.	Is the child indecisive due to poor self-confidence and self-esteem?		
15.	Does the child intrude into the personal space of others?		
16.	Is the child unaware of their own physical appearance?		
17.	Does the child make inappropriate or exaggerated use of tone and gesture?		
18.	Does the child respond aggressively to teasing?		
19.	Does the child interrupt conversations?		
20.	Does the child have noisy eating habits (this could link with verbal dyspraxia)?		
21.	Does the child have difficulty using a knife and fork, often resorting to fingers?		
22.	Is there evidence of poor posture when the child is sitting? (Girls with dyspraxia may sit with legs apart.)		
23.	Is the child sensitive to noise levels? They may be unaware that the TV is turned up loudly, for example.		
24.	Does the child have difficulties in speech (such as those experienced by children with developmental verbal dyspraxia)?		

Verbal dyspraxia checklist

	Observation	Yes	No	Comments
1.	Does the child struggle to produce spoken words?			
2.	Are certain words or phrases spoken spontaneously (automatic speech), yet the child is unable to repeat them on request (voluntary speech)?			
3.	Is the child's understanding of speech much better than their expression?			
4.	Is the child's speech hard to understand?			
5.	If more effort is required to say something, does it become difficult for the child to produce the words?			
6.	Is there difficulty in expressing consonant clusters, so that 'black' may be pronounced 'lack' and 'tree' may be pronounced 'ree'?			
7.	Are difficult consonants replaced by simpler consonants; for example 'cat' is pronounced as 'tat'?			
8.	Does the child exhibit stutter-like movements, exaggerated gestures or grimacing?			
9.	Do other children complete the sentence for the child?			
10.	Is eye contact limited due to poor self-confidence and low self-esteem?			
11.	Does the child have difficulty expressing emotions?			
12.	Is there an increase in the number of errors which is directly linked to word length and the complexity of the word?			
13.	Does the child appear to be groping for words?			
14.	Are words produced in a disorganised format?			
15.	Does speech sound slow and hesitant?			
16.	Is the problem with speech deviant rather than immature (Williams *et al.*, 1980)?			

Assessment of perceptual difficulties

It was mentioned in the last chapter that it is often difficult to determine which area of perceptual difficulty the child is experiencing. Simple activities that will help are suggested. Difficulties experienced with any of these tasks may indicate that the child has perceptual problems.

Key Stages 1 and 2

Useful activities include the following:

- Ask the children to stack a series of five 10 cm cubes on top of one another (hand–eye co-ordination).
- Ask them to place ten small pegs accurately in a pegboard (hand–eye co-ordination).
- Show the children a simple drawing of a house and ask them to copy it (form constancy).
- See if the child can identify certain animals from a full sorting tray or sort certain coloured buttons from a jar (figure–ground discrimination).
- Show the child a simple drawing of two overlapping stars and ask them to colour in each in a different colour (figure–ground discrimination).
- Ask the child to draw a picture of themselves (position in space).
- Give the child a series of 10 cm cubes and ask them to copy three-dimensional designs from a two-dimensional image (spatial relationships).
- Provide the child with an age-appropriate jigsaw and ask them to complete this independently (visual closure).

Key Stages 3 and 4

Activities for these stages include the following:

- Provide a large nut and bolt and ask the child to screw the nut onto the bolt (hand–eye co-ordination).
- Provide a series of puzzles in which the children have to track and find the exact shape although it may be presented smaller or larger than the original or positioned at a different angle (form constancy).
- Show the children pictures of shapes that are superimposed over each other and ask them to find the outlines and colour in the shapes in different colours (figure–ground discrimination).
- Ask the child to draw a picture of themselves, adding as much detail as possible (position in space).
- Ask the child to reproduce a pegboard pattern (spatial relationships).
- Ask the child to finish the mirror image of half-completed pictures (visual closure).

All of the tasks suggested can be completed relatively easily by those who do not have perceptual or motor difficulties. By observing how a child with dyspraxia attempts each exercise, it is possible to gain an idea of the area of perception that is affecting the child's performance.

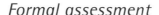

Formal assessment

There are a number of formal standardised assessments which are used primarily by occupational therapists and physiotherapists to identify motor and perceptual development. A list of these can be found in the Appendix. Many of these tests can also be utilised by teachers, especially those specialised in working with children with special educational needs.

Assessment profile

Case study: Jacob, aged 8.6 years

Jacob was born prematurely at 35 weeks' gestation following spontaneous rapid labour. His milestones were slightly delayed in that he did not crawl, preferring to bottom shuffle before getting up to walk at 18 months. Jacob walked with a wide gait, and his mother noted that when he was excited he skipped around on his tiptoes.

During his pre-school years, Jacob enjoyed pretend play and showed vivid imagination. He did not opt for sports such as football, was reluctant to use the apparatus at the park and could not ride a bike. His parents were not too concerned as they felt he was a particularly creative, imaginative child.

On entry to school he worked very hard but struggled with fine motor activities such as holding a pencil, writing and using scissors, and with constructive play such as Lego®. Physical education proved difficult as Jacob's ball skills were erratic and he was reluctant to play team games.

On entering Key Stage 1, his difficulties became more pronounced. It was clear that his problems were not related to immaturity and that more structured help would be needed. Jacob's teacher approached the SENCo with concerns particularly related to handwriting, which was poor, untidy and laboured. The SENCo provided advice about ways to support handwriting in class and Jacob was allocated some time with a teaching assistant. The teacher also ensured that, through her planning, the classroom computer was available to support Jacob during parts of the Literacy Hour and for other subject areas where it proved beneficial. In addition, Jacob was introduced to the use of IT programmes that support the writing process, such as Clicker 4 (see Appendix). This programme enables children to demonstrate their knowledge without the burden of writing ideas down.

By the end of Key Stage 1, Jacob was making some progress but still needed more support than his peers. It was decided, after consultation with his parents, that he would benefit from an individual education plan (IEP) so that specific targets could be set and his progress monitored. The school placed him on School Action; the SENCo and class teacher were responsible for the strategies to help Jacob. Jacob was involved in determining his own targets.

An example of Jacob's IEP in Year 2 is supplied. The third target was included in anticipation of the Key Stage 1 assessment.

Individual Education Plan

Name: Jacob   Date: 16. 09. 02   Class: 2b

Target	Teaching strategies and provision	Success criteria
1. Handwriting Jacob will be able to write a paragraph of text demonstrating appropriate spaces between words.	*Write from the Start* handwriting programme booklets 2-4. Teaching assistant to supervise.	Jacob will demonstrate adequate spacing between words 80 per cent of the time.
2. Co-ordination Jacob will be able to: Control scissors to cut around specific reference lines. Throw an object in a precise manner. Carry out constructive activities, especially during practical maths sessions.	Jacob will cut out from a catalogue a picture which supports his schoolwork. Teaching assistant to supervise. Target throwing will be incorporated into PE activities. Complete booklet 1 of the *Write from the Start* programme.	Cut around a 10 cm circle drawn on a piece of paper. Throw a beanbag into a bucket located 4 metres away. Stack 15 x 2 cm cubes on top of one another without their toppling.
3. Writing Jacob will be able to produce and complete a minimum of one piece of compositional writing during the term.	Provide additional time in the Literacy Hour. Teaching assistant to supervise. Provide parents with additional work to support Jacob at home.	One piece of completed writing which will be either: a simple recount linked to a topic of interest/personal experience; or: a piece of writing relating to a significant incident occurring within a story using simple settings.
Review Class teacher and SENCo meet fortnightly to review progress.		Date of next IEP update: 13/01/03

Towards the end of Key Stage 1, putting Jacob onto School Action Plus was considered as his progress slowed down. This was in part attributed to the birth of a baby sister, which had changed the home balance. This was kept in mind and reviewed in relation to his entering Key Stage 2.

As he entered Key Stage 2 expectations increased and Jacob's needs became more apparent. Fine motor activities still proved to be problematic. He became increasingly fearful of PE lessons and it was noticed that his self-confidence seemed to be decreasing. The teacher felt that there was a widening gap between Jacob's verbal skills when he joined in classroom discussions and his ability to record information in written form. Jacob rarely completed written work, in particular the composition of stories. The combined need to compose a story and write it down demonstrated Jacob's organisational and processing difficulties.

It was decided to put Jacob onto School Action Plus and gain some additional help from outside the school. In response to this, the SENCo alerted Pupil Support Services at the local education authority (LEA) and a referral was made to a local occupational therapist at the Child Development Centre. This was carried out with the approval of Jacob's parents.

The occupational therapist, together with a physiotherapist, assessed his gross and fine motor co-ordination and his visual perception skills. They also discussed his progress and difficulties with his teachers and parents before conducting a formal assessment. The results confirmed that Jacob was dyspraxic and the following strategies were implemented by health professionals:

- Participation in an after-school club known as the BCBs (balance co-ordination and body awareness). This club was run by an occupational therapist and a physiotherapist and sought to address the gross motor and visuo-spatial needs of a group of children who were all experiencing perceptuo-motor difficulties. Details of activities at this club were sent to Jacob's school and implemented in PE lessons.

- Classwork was adapted so that Jacob could focus on specific pieces of work without being overwhelmed by the volume of material. This was particularly useful in maths exercises.

- Training was given to help staff at the school understand the nature of dyspraxia and the needs of Jacob as well as how they could help to alleviate some of his difficulties.

- His parents were given a home programme which included a dressing plan and information about how to adapt his clothing to make dressing and undressing for PE easier.

- A writing programme was introduced to help Jacob master the movements and patterns needed to write effectively.

● A dictation machine was supplied for Jacob to record diaries or stories rather than writing them out, which was making Jacob anxious.

Jacob still has dyspraxia, but he is able to cope with his condition with the help of those around him and the occasional help of professionals within the Child Development Centre.

I wish they would only take me as I am.
Vincent Van Gogh

Chapter 4
Support in the classroom

Today the classroom environment is a busy place to be. Often classrooms accommodate large numbers of pupils but have limited space in which to work and store resources. In addition teachers are under considerable pressure to address the requirements of the National Curriculum. Having a child with a special need such as dyspraxia can be both confusing and frustrating. However, there are support strategies that can be put into practice in the classroom.

For children with dyspraxia there are a number of key skills that prove particularly difficult and which have a bearing on academic success. These are handwriting, numeracy and physical education. In addition children with dyspraxia will have difficulties with reading, art and craft and general organisation. Social skills may also be poor. The results of these difficulties often present emotionally and the child may be overactive and inattentive, or subdued and lacking in self-confidence.

The role of the teaching assistant

Teachers do a splendid job in striving to meet the requirements of children with special educational needs, but the additional support of a teaching assistant can never be underestimated.

For children with dyspraxia, the most effective way to help in the classroom does not necessarily involve an adult sitting alongside them and supporting them in their work. The child with dyspraxia is very conscious that their abilities are different from those of their peers and they desperately want to fit into the classroom without their weaknesses being recognised or highlighted.

How the teaching assistant helps is a vital component in successful inclusion. One of the very best ways a teaching assistant can support the child will involve time spent planning and preparing classwork.

This can include the following, for example:

- Preparing maths work so one calculation is given at a time, rather than several within a workbook.
- Instructing on the use of a dictation machine to support written work.
- Preparing specific writing activities on coloured paper.
- Obtaining a reading window to help focus when reading.
- Making sure appropriate equipment, such as an angled board to improve hand–eye co-ordination, is available when needed.
- Providing alternatives to writing, such as the use of story boards and magazine cuttings.

If the child is receiving any outside help from health care professionals such as occupational therapists, it is a good idea if possible to set up a link between the therapist and teaching assistant to share knowledge and ideas. For example, if the child is attending a special gym club, the session plans could be brought to the school and integrated by the teaching assistant into physical education lessons.

The following are strategies for the classroom which will address some of the needs of children with dyspraxia.

Handwriting

Handwriting difficulties are very common in children with dyspraxia owing to poor co-ordination and inadequate visual perception. The typical problems seen are as follows.

Hand dominance

It is important to ascertain whether the child is left or right handed. Some children often swap their pencil from one hand to another during the same activity. Children who have trouble in determining their hand preference will encounter difficulties in co-ordination and organisation. By the age of 7 years a child should have established distinct hand dominance, although some remain ambidextrous. To identify whether the child has mixed dominance or has not yet developed a preferred side, try the following activities, making a careful note of whether the left or right side of the body is used:

- Give the child a kaleidoscope (alternatively a sweet tube can be used) and ask them to peep through it.
- Whisper a joke or give the child a seashell to listen to.
- Ask the child to pick up a pencil.
- Ask the child to march like a soldier. Which foot do they lead with, right or left?
- Ask the child to kick a football.

A consistent preference should arise. If this is not the case, do not force a child to hold a pencil in their right or left hand. Instead monitor their preference over a period of time.

Some children are cross-lateral and do not seem to have a preferred hand. They should be encouraged to write as comfortably as possible and not be forced to use one hand rather than the other.

Pencil grip

It is preferable for children who are developing handwriting skills to use a pencil as that provides a measure of how much pressure they are placing through the writing instrument. This cannot be measured easily when they use a pen.

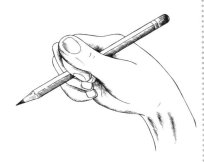

Figure 8. 'Double roll' pencil grasp, common in children with dyspraxia.

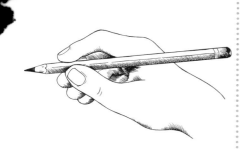

Figure 9. Dynamic tripod grip.

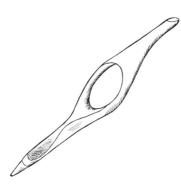

Figure 10. Ring pen.

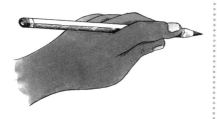

Figure 11. Altered pencil grip.

However, many children appear to hold their pencils awkwardly, which can affect their handwriting. Commonly, children with dyspraxia roll their thumb over the shaft of the pencil or roll both index and thumb over the shaft of the pencil as in Fig. 8. Both restrict pencil movement. It is important to encourage the child to hold the writing instrument in a dynamic tripod grip, which is the most effective grip to control the pencil and to see the writing (Fig. 9).

There are several ways to address these difficulties:

- Encourage the use of pencil grips such as Tri-Go grips (see Appendix). These contoured pencil grips help children develop the correct grip.
- A ring pen (Fig. 10) will ensure that the child who frequently drops items will maintain an appropriate grip on the pen (see Appendix).
- Work with the child to alter the grip, so that the pencil is held between the index and middle fingers over the top of the hand (Fig. 11).
- Manipulative activities in general will assist the child to become more aware of finger position and the complex manipulative manoeuvres required to write effectively (Naus, 2000).

If a child appears to hold a pencil awkwardly yet their handwriting is legible and the child does not complain of cramps, stiffness or aches, then there is no reason to attempt to alter the grip (Dennis and Swinth, 2001).

Physical posture

Children with dyspraxia will often be fidgety and restless in the classroom. This is due to poor auditory and visual figure–ground discrimination, inadequate proprioception, and/or a lack of integration of the senses.

Position the furniture appropriately for the child and make sure they are in the best position for working. Whilst sitting on a chair, their feet should be flat on the floor with knees and hips at 90 degrees. When seated, the height of the table should be the same as the height of the elbows when placed against the side of the body. The child's work should be placed in alignment to the child's arm, not square to the table.

Wrist position

Many children write with their wrist held off the table, which will result in writing pressure being too light and a lack of control. To reduce this habit, an angled board can be provided (Fig. 12). These can be bought from suppliers (see Writestart Desktop in Appendix) or they can be made simply from plywood, with an angle of 20 to 30 degrees depending on the child's needs. By resting the wrist on the board an appropriate position can be developed.

Pressure through the pencil

Inability to monitor pressure through the pencil results in slow, laboured writing with reduced legibility.

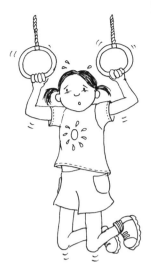

"Kelly had never imagined handwriting could be such hard work."

To address this, each child needs to be taught how to monitor their own pressure through the pencil. Pens which light up when pressure is applied can be bought and may be useful in monitoring pressure. Also, carbon paper can be used to determine the extent of pressure.

If the child has proprioceptive difficulties they will need to undertake activities to enhance their upper limb stability, such as wall press-ups and crawling.

Often older children with dyspraxia show heavy pressure and laboured handwriting. This may occur when the child has been printing for a prolonged period and is then expected to join up their writing to increase the speed of output. Often if letters have been orientated incorrectly for a prolonged period, the child finds it impossible to join them. This reduces speed at a time when the child requires increased output in preparation for secondary school.

One way to assist this is to follow a kinaesthetic approach, as advocated by the handwriting programme *Speed Up!* (see Appendix).

Letter orientation and formation

Many children with dyspraxia struggle with the orientation of letter forms and often reversals can be seen in their written work. Common errors are reversals of *b* and *d*, *f* and *t*, *p* and *q*, *m* and *w* and *n* and *u*. The letter *s* and the numbers *2*, *3*, *4*, *5*, *6*, *7* and *9* are also often inverted. This will have an effect on the child's ability to join letters correctly and will also make their work difficult to read. Reversals are common in young children, but by the age of 6 years orientation has usually been defined. With dyspraxia this is an ongoing problem and it needs to be addressed as early as possible in the child's writing career.

Orientation of letters relates to a problem with the area of perception known as position in space. One key way to help develop appropriate orientation is to introduce the child to joined (cursive) writing very early in their school life. Activities involving mirroring and completing symmetrical pictures may help. The use of *Finger Phonics* books from the Jolly Phonics series (see Appendix) may help as the letter form is indented into the book and the children can use touch to help them with the orientation of letters. Alternatively the *Write from the Start* programme (see Appendix) can help with this.

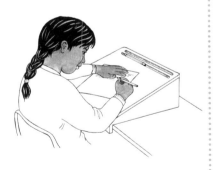

Figure 12. Provision of an angled board to improve wrist position when writing.

The following activities help children develop form constancy and directionality, which will help improve letter orientation:

- Ask the child to visualise the letter form and write this in the air with their eyes closed.
- Draw a letter on the child's back or the palm of their hand with a finger, then see if they can identify the letter form. There is evidence that this kinaesthetic approach improves handwriting (Harris and Livesey, 1992).
- Use tracker stencils to allow the child to feel the shape of the letter and the correct orientation.

○ Demonstrate clearly how a letter links onto the next, introducing cursive writing at Key Stage 1 if not earlier.

○ Introduce activities from the *Write from the Start* programme.

○ Use the Rol'n'Write alphabet to track around letter forms (see Appendix).

Writing alignment

Often children with dyspraxia will start a line of writing in the middle of the page or will start at the left-hand side and slope their writing diagonally across the page rather than track across horizontally from left to right. This is when lined paper proves essential. If this has little effect, try the following:

○ Place a coloured marker such as a star shape or bullet point in the left-hand margin and a similar point in the opposite right-hand margin so the children can see where they need to begin and finish their writing.

○ Provide raised line paper such as Stop-Go (see Appendix). This paper helps the child with ascenders and descenders, as well as with letter size and positioning.

○ Paper with different coloured lines can be produced on the computer. The children can then be encouraged to write, for example, on a blue line, then a red line and so on. As the child progresses the variety of colours can be reduced.

○ Recommended activities highlighted in the relevant section of the *Write from the Start* handwriting programme can be used to encourage correct writing alignment.

Spacing of letters and words

The child with dyspraxia has significant difficulties with spatial organisation, and this has repercussions in their handwriting. Spaces between words are frequently omitted or erratically placed. This can be frustrating for the reader as considerable time is needed to decipher the meaning.

Gross motor activities which help the children to co-ordinate have a positive effect on fine motor activities such as handwriting. In addition the following compensatory strategies may help:

○ Introducing cursive writing as soon as possible will have a positive effect on handwriting development. A programme such as *Teaching Handwriting – Continuous Cursive Handwriting and How to Teach It* may prove useful (see Appendix).

○ The child can be encouraged to leave a space between words by using a writing spacer or alternatively taught to use a finger between words.

○ Help with spacing can also be developed by asking the children to write on grid paper, placing each letter in a box.

○ The use of coloured lines when creating grids or shaded squares can also be helpful. These enable the child to focus on a particular area and place letters or words in specific locations. This is effective as many children with dyspraxia have a sensitivity to bold colour contrast such as that between

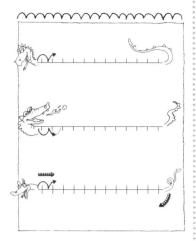

Figure 13. Example of spatial exercises taken from the *Write from the Start* programme.

black and white. Using softly coloured squares or lines provides a less stark reference point from which the child can progress.

In addition appropriate activities from the *A Hand for Spelling* series (see Appendix) and *Write from the Start* (Fig. 13) help to overcome the underlying spatial problems that can cause handwriting difficulties.

Sizing of letters and mixed upper- and lower-case letters

Children with dyspraxia often write with inconsistencies in the size of letters. This can be helped by the following strategies:

- Encouraging the use of grid paper, so that letters are placed in each space.

- Introduce activities that involve proportions. These could include looking at body proportions and mirror representations. The child could, for example, draw around a partner on a large sheet of paper and add features, the teacher pointing out size differences between parts of the body.

- Introduce the Jolly Phonics series.

- Include appropriate aspects of the *Write from the Start* handwriting programme. The difference in one child's handwriting before and after the implementation of this programme may be seen in Fig. 14.

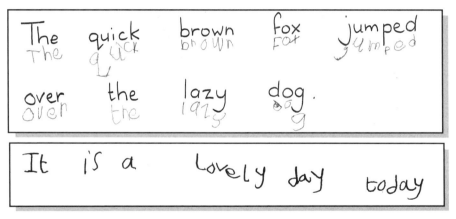

Figure 14. Sample of a child's handwriting before and after using the *Write from the Start* programme.

Speed of handwriting

There is an expectation that the speed of handwriting will increase as the child becomes more competent and confident in writing. However, for a child with dyspraxia, who struggles with this complex fine motor skill, it is often the reverse that happens: their writing slows down. This will cause the child considerable anxiety. In order to reduce this, an alternative to handwriting may be needed – such as the use of a word processor with voice-activated software.

To speed up the writing, various approaches can be adopted. The *Speed Up!* kinaesthetic handwriting programme can help to relax the child whose difficulties in handwriting have caused them to adopt a tight pencil grip and

Success always occurs in private, and failure in full view.

Anon.

produce precise, laboured handwriting. The latter stages of the *Write from the Start* programme may also help with the patterns of movement required.

Writing confidence

Children with dyspraxia typically have low self-confidence. This is especially true in relation to their handwriting. Therefore a rethink is required in terms of how to allow the child to demonstrate what they know, using a medium other than writing. Asking the children themselves was the basis of a small research project held in North Yorkshire (Addy, 1996) consisting of a group of children with dyspraxia, aged 8–12. The results revealed the creativity of children in providing solutions to their own dilemmas. They suggested the following options:

- ʼAllow me to use a dictation machine so that I can create stories and describe events. By doing this I can emphasise key issues using the inflection in my voice.ʼ
- ʼPlease test me using "pub quizzes" so I can let you know exactly what I know verbally.ʼ
- ʼPlease let me use drama and skits to convey what I know.ʼ
- ʼI struggle with writing and find it easier to tell stories and events using pictures. I cut them from comics and magazines and sequence them into stories; it ends up looking like a comic, but you can see where I am coming from.ʼ
- ʼI am experimenting at home with voice-activated programmes on my computer. This is much easier for me, and then I cross-check meanings later.ʼ

Sadly, the present educational curriculum demands considerable writing skills as evidence of a child's knowledge. Hopefully, as technology advances, the thoughts, feelings, expression and knowledge of children with dyspraxia can be presented more clearly in the future.

Numeracy

Numeracy is another area of the curriculum that causes problems for children with dyspraxia. It is not necessarily a cognitive problem but a perceptual dilemma. The cluttered material, written formation of numbers, organisation of calculations, complex language used and manipulation of physical elements can all make mathematics a complex and daunting prospect for the child with dyspraxia. Children who have the additional diagnosis of dyslexia will also have sequencing problems.

Together, difficulties in written mathematics and handwriting can lead many teachers to believe that the child has significant learning difficulties rather than difficulties specific to motor planning and perception.

To help the child with dyspraxia with numeracy, try the following suggestions.

Numbers and the number system

The following strategies may help:

- Learning how to identify and write numbers can be confusing owing to the various ways in which numbers can be written – such as *4*, 4 and *four*. One way to help is to play number Pelmanism (Pairs). To do this, make up pairs of cards with the numbers written on them in various forms, place the cards face down, then lift two cards each time and attempt to match the number pairs. A game of Snap can be played using similar cards.

- Children with dyspraxia often have difficulty in writing numbers in their correct form. El-Naggar (1996) recommends teaching the writing of numerals in groups so that certain numerals do not occur in the same group. This would mean, for example, presenting *1*, *2* and *3* initially and making sure that 3 is formed correctly before introducing *4*, *5* and *6*.

- Provide number lines. These are used to help a child progress from using fingers or counters to count, and can be graded according to ability. It is beneficial to use gross movements to demonstrate addition and subtraction, perhaps by using a large number line drawn in chalk on the playground and numbered from 1 to 10 (or more depending upon the child's learning needs). Alternatively a large coloured number line could be created from card.

- Knowledge of the sequence of numbers is a fundamental skill of counting. Many children may learn to count forwards but are unable to count backwards sequentially. Suggestions to help with this are:
  - practising days of the week and months of the year;
  - teaching rhymes;
  - patterning work using a pegboard;
  - doing jigsaws;
  - ordering tasks;
  - following recipes.

- It is important to have a range of concrete objects and mathematical apparatus in the classroom, such as Unifix® cubes and Cuisenaire® rods. These help with counting and the understanding of mathematical concepts.

- Abacuses are another useful piece of apparatus to have. They encourage the use of the index finger by moving the beads when counting. The isolation of the index finger assists with motor control and also reduces the possibility of several beads being moved together.

- Provide the children with a highlighter pen and encourage them to mark off items, so that when counting, objects and items are not recounted. Recounting is a typical feature of spatial organisation difficulties.

Calculations

The following strategies provide help with calculation:

- Provide calculators which have large clear numbers.
- Provide and use magnetic number boards to arrange sums so that they can be clearly visualised.
- Introduce audiotapes and CDs to consolidate and learn multiplication and other mathematical rules.
- Make a book of 100-number squares showing the multiplication table patterns. Encourage the child to use these for calculations which need multiplication.
- When doing work on money, attach a bead to one side of a coin to make it easier to lift (Fig. 15).

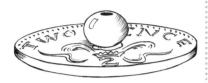

Figure 15. Adapted coin to assist in manipulation when counting money.

The language of mathematics is often complex, with different words being used to describe the same thing – for example *combine* and *add*, *subtract* and *remove*, *multiply* and *times*. Also, mathematical problems are often presented in a problem-solving manner and the interpretation of them into symbols and figures becomes complex and confusing.

It is often easier to break the information down, for example focusing on all the expressions relating to addition, such as:

- Jane has seven marbles. John has five. How many marbles do they have altogether?
- I have seven sweets. You have five. If I give you my sweets, how many would you have altogether?

Here are some more suggestions to help with calculations:

- The Pelmanism game can also be used to differentiate the symbols used in mathematics; cards can be made showing the forms of addition as well as the other calculations. Ensure that the child has fully understood a concept before moving on to a new term.
- Include practical calculations which have real-life relevance to the child. These are more easily understood.
- Encourage the children to read numbers out loud so that it is possible to check their understanding of calculation.

Recording

Often the way in which numeracy problems and examples are presented can be improved for the child with dyspraxia:

- It will help if the amount of information on a workbook page is reduced, perhaps by separating the sums. Presenting calculations one at a time reduces the amount of visual stimuli. One way in which this can be done is to provide a card window which is positioned over the page to reveal one calculation. This will improve figure–ground discrimination.

○ When photocopying, photocopy worksheets onto pastel-coloured paper to reduce the stark contrast between black and white. Alternatively, use coloured overlays to soften the visual field so that items and objects are more easily seen.

○ Provide grid paper to assist in page organisation (Fig. 16).

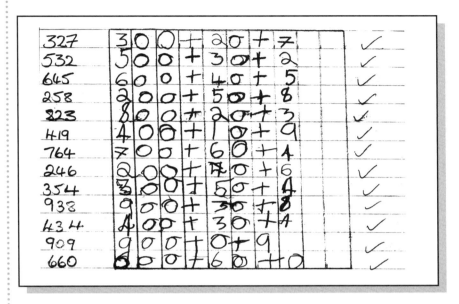

Figure 16. Use of a grid to help with spatial difficulties and improve presentation.

○ Place an arrow next to the calculation to prompt the child to the direction of calculation.

○ Similarity can also help to focus the eye. When this is applied to the layout of mathematics, it becomes clear from which direction the sum should be calculated, as can be seen in Fig. 17.

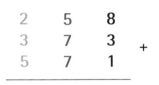

Figure 17. Use of similarity to highlight direction of calculation.

Measures, shape and space

The following strategies are suggested:

○ Check that the child has an understanding of spatial concepts. This involves the ability to recognise and use appropriate space and position concepts; for example *under*, *through*, *opposite*, *in between*. To help reinforce these terms take the child physically through the positions described; for example ask the child to sit under a table.

○ Provide rulers with a raised handle to hold them in place to aid motor control (see My First Ruler, Appendix). If these are not available, add a small blob of Blu-Tac® to either end of the base of a ruler to prevent it slipping when drawing geometric forms.

○ Use reference points or broken lines to help create a specific shape, remembering that diagonal lines are particularly difficult for children with dyspraxia. Shapes can also be created using Geoboards (see Appendix).

○ Use plastic shape stencils to help create patterns and pictures (see Attribute Blocks and Pattern Blocks, Appendix).

○ Give a physical reinforcement of certain measures. For example, measure the child's hand span and use this to approximate distances.

Other considerations

○ Some children may have difficulty with short-term memory and may not progress from the basic tactics of physically counting on fingers to retrieving strategies from memory. They continue to depend upon time-consuming physical methods. To help with this try the following:

  ○ Limit the number of sequences within instructions.
  ○ Use a multi-sensory approach with a mixture of verbal problem solving, practical problem solving and written and recorded sequences of instructions.
  ○ Limit the time spent on the subject to prevent overload.
  ○ Introduce fun tactics to ensure that the child continues to be motivated; for example memory games such as 'Mrs Brown went to town'.
  ○ Use Duplo® or Lego® as counting rods and make them into interesting models.
  ○ Encourage rote learning of tables in rhyme form.
  ○ Teach rhymes such as 'Thirty days has September' which aid memory.
  ○ For younger children teach nursery rhymes that involve numbers and sequences of numbers.

○ In order to maintain the child's attention and motivation:

  ○ Ensure that work is at an age-appropriate level.
  ○ Revisit previous work and skills.
  ○ Do not rehash previously completed work.
  ○ Allow time and set individualised programmes.
  ○ Remember that there is a need to repeat learning but beware of motivational burn-out.

Physical education

As children with dyspraxia have significant difficulties with motor planning and execution, physical education can be a stressful experience. It is also a cause of considerable low self-esteem and confidence as children often place importance on performing well in sporting activities. The following suggestions will help children with dyspraxia develop their visual perception and motor co-ordination.

Activities for weak shoulder and hip stability

Many children with dyspraxia have an unstable shoulder and hip girdle. This can be seen when you ask a child to balance on all four limbs. In this position, ask the child to raise an opposite arm and leg (Fig. 18). If the child appears unstable or topples this indicates a weakness.

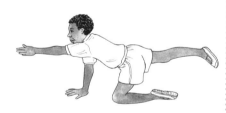

Figure 18. Four-point kneel with opposite arm and leg raised.

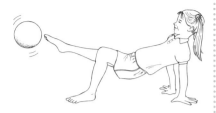

Figure 19. Position required to play crab football.

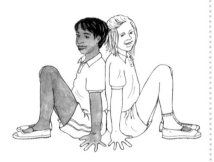

Figure 20. Resistance race with children back to back.

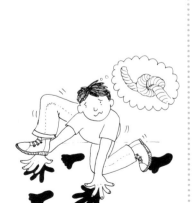

Shoulder instability will produce poor co-ordination for writing and activities such as fastening buttons, scissor work, sewing and construction. Hip instability will affect walking, running, jumping and hopping as well as influencing posture when the children are sitting or standing. Many children with significant problems in this area will prefer to sit and seem lethargic. They may also be prone to becoming overweight because their activity is limited. It is important that activities to improve hip and shoulder stability are included within physical education lessons. These could include the following:

○ Crab football, in which a crab position is held and the children attempt to kick the ball towards a goal (Fig. 19).

○ Floor football. Here the children are sitting on the floor, either cross-legged or with straight legs, in two teams with a goal at either end. Once positioned they must not move their bottoms from the floor and must attempt to push the ball towards the goal using their hands only. The ball must not be held and must remain less than 0.5 metres from the floor. This takes considerable upper limb effort, while promoting pelvic stability.

○ Port/Starboard. This game involves a pretend ship. The children are given ship commands and follow them to stay in the game. 'Port' requires running to the right, 'Starboard' to the left. Additional instructions are 'Scrub the deck', whereupon the children pretend to scrub the deck on their hands and knees; 'Man overboard', whereupon they balance on one leg; 'Rats on the deck', which requires hopping from one foot to the other; 'Climb the rafters', in which the children pretend to climb a pole, and 'Walk the gangplank', which involves a two-footed jump.

○ Resistance race. This involves sitting with legs straight in front, feet touching a partner's. The child tries to push their partner forward using their arms, keeping their legs straight. The same idea can be tried with the children back to back and trying to push with feet rather than hands (Fig. 20).

○ Bottom-walking competitions.

○ Hand and feet obstacle course. Working in small teams of approximately six children, each child draws around their hands and feet. These can then be cut out or used as drawings. Each team sticks the feet and hands onto the floor, forming an obstacle course for the other teams. Rival team members must cross the room by placing their hands and feet on appropriate stencils in order to cross the room safely and quickly.

○ Frozen beanbag. Provide everyone playing the game with a beanbag. This is balanced on the children's heads. The children move around the room either to music or to instructions. If a child's beanbag falls off they are frozen and cannot move until another person picks up their beanbag for them and replaces it on their head. The child picking up the beanbag must do so without their own beanbag falling off their head. The winner is the person who has helped to return the most beanbags in a given time.

Activities for spatial organisation

Perceptual problems may affect performance in physical education. Problems with spatial organisation can cause particular difficulties for children with dyspraxia. The following are some activities that can help:

- Clumps. The children walk or gently run around the room. When the teacher shouts a number, a group or clump containing that number should be formed. For example, if the number called is 5, the children should form groups of 5. If any children are left over, they should form a group themselves near the teacher.

- Beanbag target games. Examples include throwing beanbags into hoops or buckets, or simply over lines.

- How many steps? Set the children a target, for example a chair in the room. They are asked the question 'How many steps do you think it would take to walk to that chair?' The child guesses, then carries out the task to see how close they were. This helps to monitor distances.

- Obstacle courses. Set obstacle courses of varying difficulty that children have to find their way around.

- Music and movement techniques such as Dalcroze Eurythmics and Laban dance (see Appendix).

- Encourage the children to play bowls or boccia. This will help them develop judgement of space.

Activities to improve hand–eye co-ordination

Many sports activities and games require effective hand–eye co-ordination. In order to develop these skills allow the children to progress through activities which will build up their ability to respond to a moving object by a hand action. The following may help:

- Provide the children with a mark at which they will stand to throw a beanbag. The aim is to throw the beanbag from the mark over lines of increasing distance and into hoops and buckets at various distances. Progress to throwing other objects graduated in weight. Start with a heavy ball as these tend to move more slowly, and progress to a tennis ball which has considerably more bounce.

- Practise throwing one object to another child, starting with a balloon which will move slowly and progressing to a beanbag and then a variety of balls.

- Create a personal target box. The children take a cardboard box and cut out shapes large enough to accept a beanbag. They can then practise target throwing and can swap targets with other class members.

- Encourage bat and ball skills by using a swing ball. The child can practise at home before attempting to use a bat and ball at school.

- Practise catching a ball using a Velcro Scatch with the paddle placed on the palm of the hand.

○ When learning tennis, start with a racquet with a shorter handle than usual, or use a heavier ball, which travels more slowly than a tennis ball.

○ Practise the skills needed for hockey by initially playing 'funny hockey' using rolled-up pieces of newspaper made into 'sticks' approximately 45 cm long. Reduce the number of players in each team and the size of the court. Gradually expand the length of stick and move onto plastic ones before attempting real hockey sticks.

Activities to develop eye–foot co-ordination

Football is a very popular sport. Often children who have difficulties with eye–foot co-ordination will have extreme difficulty playing, whether in a kick-around on the school playing field or under formal instruction.

A task-centred approach can be helpful in enabling children to kick a ball in a forward direction. Repeated practice of key kicking skills can enable the child to build up the skills required to kick the ball, even if they do that from a static position only. The following may help in developing eye–foot co-ordination:

○ Use a Kik a Flik (see Appendix). This is an ingenious game in which a ball is placed on the end of a short seesaw. When one end is stamped the ball flies into the air towards the child, who attempts to catch it. This is an excellent activity to teach children how to monitor pressure through their lower limbs.

○ Place a ball in a small hoop. The child moves around the hoop touching the ball with different parts of the feet, but keeping the ball in the hoop (Russell, 1988).

○ Practise kicking the ball forward to a goal from a sitting position.

○ Try rolling the ball towards the child before they kick it. This reduces the need for the child to judge the distance from the ball, which is another complex skill required to play football.

○ Vary the weight and size of the balls used in kicking and football activities.

Activities for visual figure–ground discrimination

Many children with dyspraxia will find the physical education environment very daunting due to the expanse of space and the number of people operating at various speeds within it. This can be overwhelming and cause the child either to cling to the wall or to run around the room with no real consideration for others or appreciation of appropriate space. It is important to try to control this and to help the children develop an appreciation of space.

○ If the area is very large, restrict its size by cordoning off parts using gym benches, tape or chalk.

○ Where it is possible, provide the children with their own space, for example by giving them a mat or a hoop to work in.

○ Where appropriate, carry out activities that do not involve the whole class moving together, especially if the class is particularly large.

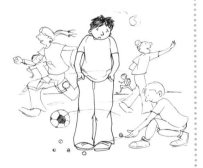

"Many children with dyspraxia will find the physical education environment very daunting."

- Teach the child clues such as 'touch and freeze' for certain movements. For example, when a certain movement is required the child knows they should start when their shoulder is touched lightly. When the shoulder is touched again the child must become as still as a statue.

- As far as possible, remove any unnecessary clutter from the environment.

- Brain Gym® is a movement-based programme consisting of 26 easy and enjoyable targeted activities that are claimed to bring about rapid and often dramatic improvements in areas such as concentration, memory, reading, writing, organising, listening and physical co-ordination. It works by developing the brain's neural pathways through movement which stimulates the sensory, auditory and proprioceptive systems (see Appendix).

Reading

Children with dyspraxia will often start school with relatively good reading abilities, especially if they have been taught using a multi-sensory phonetic approach to letter recognition such as that advocated through Jolly Phonics (see Appendix).

However, as reading progresses, deterioration may be noted. This is primarily due to the increased number of words on a page and the reduction in the size of the letters. The child with dyspraxia will be required to concentrate in order to focus on the print, and will often say that the print 'bounces' or 'blurs'. Distractions will make it more difficult to focus on reading. In order to help alleviate this, try the following:

- Reduce the amount of information on the page by covering the text on the line above or below that being read. Reading windows can be obtained which will highlight just one line of reading at a time (see Appendix).

- Enlarge the letter size by using a photocopier or a magnifying glass.

- Photocopy the print onto a pastel-coloured background as this reduces the intensity of contrast between black on white. A coloured overlay can also help to reduce the effect of black print on a white background.

- Some children who find reading particularly difficult may have Irlen Syndrome or Scotopic Sensitivity Syndrome. Children with this condition are particularly sensitive to light; contrasting colours such as black text on white paper will appeared blurred. It may be helpful to have a colorimeter assessment undertaken by an optician or hospital ophthalmic department. This will determine the best colour contrast for reading and give guidance for buying spectacles with tinted lenses.

- Try to read with the child in a quiet, distraction-free part of the classroom to maximise concentration level and encourage reading for short bursts.

- Highlight key words or themes from a book with a highlighter pen to enable the child to identify the key aspects of the story. Sometimes children are so absorbed in reading each word that the meaning or joy of the text is lost. Highlighting certain words ensures that the key components of the story are focused on.

Adversity causes some men to break; others to break records.

William A. Ward

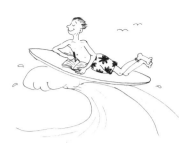

"Provide an angled board."

○ Provide an angled board with an angle of approximately 20 degrees. This will optimise the child's posture and help to channel the visual field (see Writestart Desktop, in Appendix).

○ Use easy-to-read fonts such as Comic Sans.

In addition to the difficulties listed above, children with verbal dyspraxia may have specific difficulties relating to reading, owing to poor phonological expression. Advice can be sought from the child's speech and language therapist, who will recommend particular ways to help the child to read.

Art and craft

It is a fallacy to think that children with dyspraxia lack creativity and imagination. It is also not true that they will shy away from art and craft activities owing to their poor hand–eye co-ordination. Children with dyspraxia often have wonderful ideas but may struggle with many conventional art activities.

It is worth bearing in mind that certain activities will be particularly difficult. Reproducing still-life drawings, for example, may prove problematic for those who struggle to see in three dimensions. Self-portraits will be affected by a poor body schema and pen and ink reproductions may be influenced by poor hand–eye co-ordination and motor control. However, there are less conventional ways of producing creative pieces of work.

The child with dyspraxia should be able to access the National Curriculum in relation to this area but may need additional equipment to help them in producing creative work. The following are worth consideration:

○ Encourage the use of photography, especially using digital imagery.

○ Provide spring-loaded scissors (see Appendix).

○ Encourage abstract art such as batik rather than representational art such as still-life drawings.

○ Encourage the use of computer design programmes, such as those related to the Art Attack series (see Appendix).

○ Use thin Dycem® matting, which will keep paper in position (see Appendix).

○ Apply the techniques suggested in the section on handwriting (pages 37–42) to develop pencil and crayon control.

Social skills and communication

For many children with dyspraxia, social skills are often impaired due to poor motor and perceptual organisation (Willoughby *et al.*, 1995). This can affect self-esteem and self-confidence, which in turn can affect social relationships and behaviour. Sometimes children may not be aware of the influence of their behaviour on others, and this may lead to social rejection and isolation.

Some children with dyspraxia may have the additional problem of verbal dyspraxia. Poor speech will inevitably affect social relationships. The characteristics of children with verbal dyspraxia are distinct; for ways to help with this area see page 53.

Children with dyspraxia may have characteristics that are out of sync with usual social behaviour. One of the most frustrating facets of this is that often the child is ridiculed and occasionally bullied because of behaviour which they are either unaware of or do not know how to change. The child's self-confidence is likely to be dented by the gibes of their peers. It is important that, when identifying social behaviours, the child's abilities are highlighted as well as their difficulties; attributes can be rewarded and praised while other aspects of social conduct are addressed.

The following are examples of games which can be used to promote various social skills:

● *Line up.* The class is divided into two groups. The teacher calls out a category such as 'Height' and each team must arrange themselves accordingly – for height with the tallest at one end, the shortest at the other. The team who are organised first are the winners. Other categories that can be used include age, hair colour and distance of home from school. This encourages team work and organisational skills.

● *Non-verbal line-up.* This follows the game described above, but class members are not allowed to use verbal communication to organise the group. This encourages children to consider alternative means of communication.

● *Who in the group?* The key rule of this game is that only positive things can be asked. The children sit in a small circle of 6–8. One child is selected to sit in the middle. Members of the group take it in turns to ask the person in the centre a question which must start with the phrase 'Who in the group'. For example, 'Who in the group would you most like to go on holiday with you?' 'Who in the group would you like by your side if you were ill?' The child in the centre then chooses a group member in response to each question. They are encouraged not to select the same person twice. When everyone has asked a question, a different child goes into the centre instead. This game encourages positive feedback and leads children to think about the personal qualities of each group member.

● *How are you feeling?* The children sit in a small circle. One member goes out of the room. The remaining children are given a card naming an emotion. The child returns to the group and asks the other members a few questions. They answer in the manner of the card; for example angrily, nervously, or apprehensively. The child who left the room tries to guess the emotion being shown. This game encourages the initiation of conversation and sensitivity towards the feelings of others.

- *The toast burned!* This game involves children working in groups of 3. One member makes a statement such as 'The toast burned'. The next child suggests a reason why – such as 'because the toaster was too hot' – and the third child formulates a solution: 'so everyone had charcoal for breakfast'. This encourages problem-solving skills and turn taking.

- *Conversational rules.* Here the children are divided into small groups of 6–8. Two members in each group are given a series of cards describing conversational mistakes; for example 'talks too fast', 'no eye contact' and 'interrupts conversations'. The pair then have a conversation incorporating these mistakes. Other group members must decide which conversational rules are being broken. These are discussed with the teacher. This game encourages sensitivity and discussion about the unspoken rules of good conversation.

Additional ideas for encouraging social skills are included in the books listed in the Appendix.

To address some of the practical difficulties which affect appearance and have an impact on peer relationships, the following strategies are useful:

- Provide wet wipes to improve hygiene after using the toilet.

- Provide a small hand mirror so that the child can check their appearance after eating.

- Place a mirror on one wall to the side of the toilet so that the child can check their clothing is in order after using the toilet.

- Consider the use of a Splayd. This is a piece of cutlery that combines a fork, spoon and knife (see Appendix).

Verbal dyspraxia

Some children with dyspraxia may have particular communication problems associated with verbal dyspraxia.

Unlike many other aspects of dyspraxia, verbal dyspraxia does not respond easily to treatment and requires the continued support of a speech and language therapist. This is a complex condition which requires considerable patience and understanding. Lax oral musculature may also influence feeding and oral hygiene and eating habits may be poor. The advice offered by the speech and language therapist will be invaluable. Further guidance is available from the website www.apraxia-kids.org.

The following strategies can be implemented both in the school and at home:

- Children with verbal dyspraxia tend to become more frustrated than others. They are often able to communicate a message spontaneously, but when asked to repeat a statement or question – or if put on the spot – will not be able to communicate effectively. The best way to help is to reduce the pressure on the child.

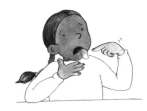

"Recognise when a child needs a break from speech-related activities."

- Encourage the child to undertake low-pressure verbal activities such as singing repetitive songs like 'Ten green bottles'. Singing helps to develop a sense of verbal rhythm.

- If the child is struggling, give them an option to cue the correct response. Try not to complete sentences for the child.

- Encourage spontaneous expression. Automatic speech comes more naturally than that requiring conscious effort. It is better for a child to utter two or three spontaneous words than to copy a sentence of seven words.

- Encourage the use of alternative forms of speech such as gestures, sign language, body language and pictures.

- Recognise when a child needs a break from speech-related activities.

- Remember to give the child choices rather than demanding a statement – for example, 'Do you want to read or to complete your writing now?'

- Technology advice may be offered by non-profit-making organisations such as AbilityNet, who offer impartial recommendations regarding computer software, adapted technology or communication devices and SEMERC (see Appendix).

- Encourage appropriate pitch by using activities which distinguish tone and volume – for example read with inflection and intonation, tell jokes with exaggerated expression and take turns to read lines from simple plays.

- Use musical instruments to develop pitch, with loud beats matching emphasised pitch and softer beats reflecting more subtle tones. Musical instruments can also be used to beat out the number of syllables in a word.

- Play games which encourage variations in speech volume – for example Chinese whispers.

- Work on sequencing skills using games and songs relating to the days of the week and the months of the year.

- Use fun raps and chants to promote spontaneous speech (Crary, 1993).

Classroom adaptations

There are several tactics which teachers and parents can use to assist the child with dyspraxia. These include the following:

- The classroom should not be overstimulating. Visual stimuli can easily overwhelm the child, especially if they have visual figure–ground discrimination difficulties. If it is not possible to achieve this, a quiet area will help the child to focus.
- If possible, the child should sit facing forward in class, near the front. Try to ensure that the child is sitting in the correct posture, fully on the chair with their feet on the ground and not bent over or resting on the desk.
- Reduce noise and distractions when giving the child detailed instructions to aid their auditory discrimination and their short-term memory.
- Allow the child time to organise and plan their activities, especially when writing a story or longer piece of work.
- Be aware that the child may use strategies to avoid carrying out tasks they find difficult.
- Try to praise at least one piece of work each day.
- Remember to ask for verbal responses as well as written work. This will allow the child to indicate how much they really know.
- Show appreciation of the things they are good at.
- Introduce joined writing as early as possible to develop fluency and spaces between words when writing.
- Worksheets should ideally be printed on pastel-coloured paper rather than on white.
- Try to vary teaching approaches and methods. Practical learning through demonstration, experimentation and hands-on work helps children with dyspraxia.
- Give a small amount of verbal or written information at a time and reduce the volume of words when giving dictation.
- If the child has poor planning and organisational skills, break each task into smaller bits. Provide strategies for them to organise themselves and their work.
- In physical education, as much as possible do activities that the child can join in with.
- Allow more time for undressing and dressing before and after physical education.
- Children will be better at reproducing drawings for art if a photograph of the object is used rather than the actual object. This applies also to self-portraits.
- Provide guidance about spatial concepts when dressing for physical education; that is remind the child what the following are: *top, bottom, inside, front, left* and *right*.
- Motor skills programmes such as Madeleine Portwood's exercise plan may help to improve the child's motor co-ordination (Portwood, 1999).
- Be aware that difficulties may manifest themselves again, especially during sudden growth spurts.

Chapter 5
Final questions

Whom can I turn to for further advice?

The strategies recommended in this book are designed to give teachers ideas to try at school in order to help children with dyspraxia help themselves. However, the needs of children with dyspraxia can be complex and there may be occasions where further specialist advice is needed.

This is where occupational therapists, physiotherapists, and speech and language therapists (if the child has verbal dyspraxia) can help. Psychologists and peripatetic teachers of special educational needs also offer considerable guidance.

These professionals tend to be in short supply. Therefore it is important to understand and support the child with dyspraxia using the aforementioned suggestions as far as possible, seeking specialist input and intervention only when necessary.

Therapists can be contacted via the child's general practitioner or directly via the local Child Development Centre based in a hospital.

The child's school will often have a named educational psychologist or special educational needs advisor.

General information on the role of these professionals is given below.

Occupational therapists

Occupational therapists are concerned with the child's functional skills. They aim towards practical independence in all areas of the child's life. They will work with issues that are a concern at home, such as dressing, undressing, social skills and play. At school they will work to enable each child to maximise their academic potential. Occupational therapists will consider perceptual and motor skills in particular, providing advice, consultations and interventions. Particular help is offered with fine motor control and perception in relation to handwriting.

Many occupational therapists are qualified to offer sensory integration, a specialised therapy which helps children with dyspraxia to integrate and order the dysfunctional sensory information they receive from their environment.

Physiotherapists

Physiotherapists work to maximise a child's physical potential and will focus on gross motor co-ordination, particularly in relation to physical education. They will advise on how to develop skills, and will also advise on special footwear, if needed.

Speech and language therapists

The speech and language therapist can offer specialist advice for children with verbal dyspraxia, at both school and home, to enhance their ability to articulate efficiently.

Psychologists

In situations where how much of a mismatch there is between the child's functional skills and cognition is unclear, the educational psychologist can offer objective assessments and considered advice to identify the child's areas of strength and weakness. They can then provide advice on strategies to help the child maximise their cognitive ability.

Clinical psychologists may become involved if the child's behaviour or emotional well-being is a concern.

Special educational needs advisor

Special needs advisors have experience of a range of childhood conditions which impinge on education and are able to suggest appropriate strategies to help the individual child meet the requirements of the National Curriculum. They have the advantage of being qualified teachers who appreciate the demands placed on both the child and their teachers in the school setting.

Parents

Never forget the value of each child's parents. I have learned more about dyspraxia from parents than from any medical or educational training I have had.

Sometimes it is easy to forget that the parents spend more time with their child than anyone else does. They can provide guidance about what makes the child happy, sad, agitated, frustrated, demoralised and content. Often they have had to discover strategies to manage at home.

In a busy working environment, it is not always possible to keep up with the latest research or interventions in relation to dyspraxia. Parents can. Many invest their physical and emotional resources in helping their child. Information from parents can be a way of keeping up with even international discussions regarding dyspraxia.

Is it important to get a diagnosis?

In terms of how to help the child, it is important that their needs are fully identified and understood. This will require comprehensive assessment including fine and gross motor co-ordination and visual perception.

Many parents may have had years of frustration, knowing that their child was not functioning as well as other children and wanting to know why. Having a diagnosis can relieve much frustration but the application of a label can have

consequences for the child's inclusion at school, particularly with respect to peer relationships. Consider the debate 'To label or not to label; that is the question?' (Addy and Dixon, 1999).

Should the child with dyspraxia be statemented?

In a study of 454 children with dyspraxia (Pullen, 1997), 54.9 per cent of the children attending state mainstream school had a statement of their educational needs.

In some cases, statementing may help a child with dyspraxia, but application for formal assessment should be considered very carefully. By highlighting their weaknesses through the statementing procedure, psychological damage may be done.

The school should weigh up the argument in the case of each individual child and answer the following questions:

- Can we identify the child's needs?
- Can we provide a programme which will help to meet their needs?
- Can we seek advice from health care professionals regarding the best approach to use with them?

These and other issues need to be thought through before a decision is taken to apply for a statement. The most important thing is to consider what would most help the child. Often it is far more constructive for the teacher to seek advice from relevant professionals regarding how best to address the child's needs in the classroom.

Are there any associations that offer support and help?

The Dyspraxia Foundation is a charitable trust devoted to supporting children with dyspraxia and those involved in their care and well-being. There are local representatives all over the country (see Appendix).

There are also associations that can help with more specific needs, a few of which are mentioned below.

Handwriting

The Handwriting Interest Group specialises in examining all types of writing needs. It draws together evidence about relevant writing equipment, gadgets and pens, styles of writing, issues of speed and examination techniques. The information is presented in an annual journal. The association also has an interactive website and an expert group of professionals to answer specific questions (see Appendix).

People with dyspraxia are like salmon trying to get up a waterfall. If they can't do it at first, they have to keep on trying so that they can survive . . .

Natalie Leer

Physical education

One helpful association is the Youth Sport Trust (see Appendix).

What about the future?

I have recently seen three students with dyspraxia being awarded high-class honours in a degree course in professional health studies. They struggled with many aspects of their learning at school. However, with the help of personally adopted strategies there are few limits to what a person with dyspraxia can achieve. The main constraint is the psychological damage that may occur over many years of underachieving, failing and being misunderstood. Hopefully, with the current increase in enlightened professionals this will not be as common in the future.

A final thought

The hidden word

In the Literacy Hour at school today
I heard a new word, dyspraxia, they say.
I don't understand, what does this word
    mean?
Does it make a noise? Is it something I've
    seen?
Can you touch it? How does it feel?
Maybe it's something you have with your
    meal!

This boy in my class doesn't write very well,
'You're just slow and lazy,' the teachers
    did yell.
'I'm tired of shouting – you must pay
    attention,
If you don't work harder you'll get a
    detention.'
This made the boy feel worthless and sad,
Then at playtime his behaviour was bad.

The other kids brag, 'We can do more
    than him!'
Teasing, name calling, stupid and dim.
The bullies say he's got special needs,
Is this a germ or some kind of disease?
Some say he's clumsy, some say he's thick,
I wouldn't say it – he's got muscles like
    a brick.

The boy in my class, well he's different
    you see,
He's bendy and floppy when it comes to PE.
He sticks out his tongue and closes one eye,
When the ropes are brought out, he's quiet
    and shy.
His mother, she looks down and so worried,
She spoke to the teacher because he was
    bullied.

We had a great time at school today,
Happy and laughing at work and at play.
The bullies were told it was wrong to tease,
So be kind and considerate and aim to please.
The boy was confident and tried his best,
He's bright, he did well in the SATs test.

The teacher, she gave him a smiley face,
His sad face disappeared without a trace.
We now understand the meaning of this
    word,
It was our behaviour that was absurd.
Now he has friends and they think he's
    fantastic,
The boy in my class is the one who's
    dyspraxic.

By kind permission of Cherry Bullimore

Children with dyspraxia have a condition that is not physically visible and that is hard to understand, the results of which will have a significant bearing on their academic attainment and well-being.

'Come to the edge,' he said. They said 'We are afraid.' 'Come to the edge,' he said. They came. He pushed them . . . and they flew.

Guillaume Apollinaire

It is hoped that this book has enabled each reader to obtain some insight into how frustrating and confusing the world can be to a child with dyspraxia and to use this understanding to select strategies which will help each child fulfil their potential. Children with dyspraxia do not all have the same characteristics, or struggle with the same dilemmas; each is a unique individual with strengths and abilities waiting to be discovered.

It is important that teachers appreciate the psychological and social effects of this complex condition for the child, understand why they behave as they do, are sensitive to their struggles with many areas of the curriculum, and are aware of their vulnerability in developing appropriate peer relationships.

The child's experiences, both positive and negative, will shape their future. Insight into and knowledge about their condition will help each child to look back on their education as a positive and rich experience.

Appendix

Main suppliers

Ann Arbor Publishers Limited
Tel: 01668 214460
www.annarbor.co.uk

LDA
Tel: 0845 120 4776
www.LDAlearning.com

Nottingham Rehab Supplies
Tel: 0845 120 4522
www.nrs-uk.co.uk

Practical resources and recommended programmes

Where no contact details are shown, they will be found in the list of main suppliers above.

A Hand for Spelling
Programme by Charles Cripps which teaches spelling and handwriting together.
LDA

Art Attack
Europress. Available from R-E-M
Tel: 01458 254700
www.r-e-m.co.uk

Clicker 4
Crick Software Ltd
Tel: 01604 671691
www.cricksoft.com

Dycem® Matting
Nottingham Rehab Supplies

Geoboards
LDA

Jolly Phonics
Tel: 020 8501 0405
www.jollylearning.co.uk

Kik a Flik
LDA

My First Ruler
LDA

Pattern Blocks
LDA

Reading Window
LDA

Ring Pen
Nottingham Rehab Supplies

Rol'n'Write
LDA

Speed Up!
A kinaesthetic handwriting programme by Lois Addy.
LDA

Splayd
Nottingham Rehab Supplies

Spring-loaded scissors
To help with the co-ordination necessary for effective cutting.
Galt Educational
Tel: 08451 20 30 05
www.galt-educational.co.uk

Stop-Go Right-Line® Paper
Taskmaster Ltd
Tel: 0116 270 4286
www.taskmasteronline.co.uk

Teaching Handwriting – Continuous Cursive Handwriting and How to Teach It
Oldfield School, Chiltern Road, Maidenhead, Berkshire, SL6 1XA
Tel: 01628 621750

Tri-Go Grips
Uniquely designed contoured pencil grips.
LDA

Write from the Start
A perceptuo-motor approach to handwriting by Lois Addy and Ion Teodorescu.
LDA

Writestart Desktop
Angled board set at 20 degrees, with non-slip surface.
LDA

Useful addresses and websites

AbilityNet
Tel: 0800 269545
www.abilitynet.org.uk

Apraxia-Kids
www.apraxia-kids.org

Brain Gym®
www.braingym.org

Dalcroze Eurythmics
The Dalcroze Society, 100 Elborough Street, London, SW18 5DL
http://home.freeuk.net/dalcroze/dalcrozeright.html

The Dyspraxia Foundation
8 West Alley, Hitchin, Hertfordshire, SG5 1EG
Tel: 01462 454986
www.dyspraxiafoundation.org.uk

National Handwriting Association
12 Isis Avenue, Bicester, Oxfordshire, OX26 2GS
www.nha-handwriting.org.uk

Laban
Creekside, London, SE8 3DZ
Tel: 020 8691 8600
www.laban.org

Harcourt Assessment
Halley Court, Jordan Hill, Oxford, OX2 8EJ
Tel: 01865 888188
www.harcourt-uk.com

SEMERC
Granada Learning, The Chiswick Centre, 414 Chiswick High Road, London, W4 5TF
Tel: 0161 827 2719
www.semerc.com

Youth Sport Trust
Sir John Beckwith Centre for Sport, Loughborough University, Loughborough, Leicestershire, LE11 3TU
Tel: 0150 922 6600
www.youthsporttrust.org

Formal assessments

Developmental Test of Visual–Motor Integration (VMI), 4th edition.
Available from Ann Arbor Publishers Limited, see address on page 61.

Motor-free Visual Perception Test–3 (MVP–3).
Available from Ann Arbor Publishers Limited.

Movement Assessment Battery for Children (Movement ABC).
Available from Harcourt Assessment, see address left.

Test of Visual Perception Skills (non-motor) (TVPS[n-m]-R) and (TVPS[n-m]UL-R).
Available from Ann Arbor Publishers Limited.

Social skills

These resources offer help with developing social skills.

Bond, T. (1986) *Games for Social and Life Skills.* Nelson Thornes.

Mosley, J. and Sonnet, H. (2003) *101 Games for Social Skills.* LDA.

Remocker, A.J. and Storch, E.T. (1999) *Actions Speaks Louder: A Handbook of Non-verbal Group Techniques.* 6th Edition. Churchill Livingstone.

Schroeder, A. (1996) *Socially Speaking.* LDA.

Schroeder, A. (2001) *Time to Talk.* LDA.

Schroeder, A. (2003) *The Socially Speaking Game.* LDA.

Schroeder, A. (2005) *The Time to Talk Game.* LDA.

References

Addy, L.M. (1995) An Evaluation of a Perceptuo-motor Handwriting Programme. York University. Unpublished master's thesis.

Addy, L.M. (1996) Unlocking the will to learn. www.letmelearn.com

Addy, L.M. and Dixon, G. (1999) To Label or Not to Label; That is the Question. *British Journal of Therapy and Rehabilitation,* vol. 5, no. 8.

American Psychiatric Association (APA) (1994) Diagnostic and Statistical Manual of Mental Disorders. 4th edition. Washington DC: APA.

Ayres, J. (1979) *Sensory Integration and the Child.* Los Angeles: Western Psychological Services.

Brooks-Gunn, J., Liaw, F.W. and Klebanov, P.K. (1992) Effects of Early Intervention on Cognitive Function of Low Birth Weight Pre-term Infants. *Journal of Pediatrics,* vol. 120, no. 3, 350–9.

Cermak, S.A. (1991) Somatodyspraxia. Cited in Fisher, A.G., Murray, E.A. and Bundy, A. *Sensory Integration: Theory and Practice.* Philadelphia: F.A. Davis Co.

Crary, M. (1993) *Developmental Motor Speech Disorders.* Whurr Publishers.

Cratty, B.J. (1979) *Perceptual and Motor Development in Infants and Children.* Prentice-Hall.

Cratty, B.J. (1994) *Clumsy Child Syndromes: Descriptions, Evaluations, and Remediations.* Harwood Academic.

Dennis, J.L. and Swinth, Y. (2001) Pencil Grasp and Children's Handwriting Legibility during Different-length Writing Tasks. *American Journal of Occupational Therapy,* vol. 55, no. 2, 175–183.

El-Naggar, O. (1996) *Specific Difficulties in Mathematics: A Classroom Approach.* NASEN

Gillberg, C. (1995) *Clinical Child Neuropsychiatry.* New York: Cambridge University Press.

Grant, L. and Watter, P. (1998) Ability to Copy Hand Positions at 10 and 12 Years of Age. *New Zealand Journal of Physiotherapy,* vol. 26, no.1, 21–5.

Gubbay, S. (1975) *The Clumsy Child: A Study of Developmental Apraxia and Agnosic Apraxia.* London: W.B. Saunders Company Ltd.

Harris, S.J. and Livesey, D.J. (1992) Improving Handwriting through Kinaesthetic Sensitivity Practice. *Australian Occupational Therapy Journal,* vol. 39, no.1, 23.

Henderson, S.E. (1993) Motor Development and Minor Handicap. In Kalverboer, A.F., Hopkins, B. and Gueze, R. *Motor Development in Early and Later Childhood. Longitudinal Approaches.* Cambridge: Cambridge University Press, 286–306.

Henderson, S.E. and Hall, D. (1982) Concomitants of Clumsy Children in Young School Children. *Developmental Medicine and Child Neurology,* no. 24, 448–60.

Hill, B. (2003) 10 most asked questions about children with developmental verbal dyspraxia. *www.dyspraxia.com.au/articles*

Johnstone, O., Short, H. and Crawford, J. (1987) Poorly Co-ordinated Children: A Survey of 95 Cases. *Childcare, Health and Development,* vol. 13, no. 6, 361–76.

Laszlo, J. and Bairstow, P. (1985) *Perceptual-motor Behaviour: Developmental Assessment and Therapy.* London: Holt, Rinehart, Winston.

Laszlo, J., Bairstow, P.J., Bartrip, J. and Rolfe. U.T (1988) Clumsiness or Perceptuo-motor Dysfunction? Cited in Colley, A.M. and Beech, R. *Cognition and Action in Skilled Behaviour.* Amsterdam: North Holland.

Lee, M. and French, J. (1994) *Dyspraxia – A Handbook for Therapists.* Association of Paediatric Chartered Physiotherapy Publications UK.

Losse, A. *et al.* (1991) Clumsiness in Children – Do they Grow out of it? A Ten Year Follow-up Study. *Developmental Medicine and Child Neurology,* vol. 33, no. 1, 55–68.

Maeland, A. (1992) Identification of Children with Motor Co-ordination Problems. *Adapted Physical Activity Quarterly,* vol. 9, no. 4.

Naus, J.M. (2000) A World of Manipulatives to Boost Handwriting Skills. *Teaching Exceptional Children,* March/April, 64–70.

Padsman, J.W., Rotteveel, J.J. and Maassen, B. (1998) Neurodevelopmental Profile in Low-risk Pre-term Infants at 5 Years of Age. *European Journal of Paediatric Neurology,* vol. 2, no. 1, 7–17.

Portwood, M. (1999) *Developmental Dyspraxia: Identification and Intervention. A Manual for Parents and Professionals.* London: David Fulton Publishers.

Pullen, T. (1997) *Member's Questionnaire. Dyspraxia Annual Review.*

Russell, J.P. (1988) *Graded Activities for Children with Motor Difficulties.* Cambridge: Cambridge University Press.

Williams, R., Packman,A., Ingham, R. and Rosenthal, J. (1980) Clinician Agreement on Behaviours that Identify Developmental Articulatory Dyspraxia. *Australian Journal of Human Communication Disorder,* vol. 8, 16–26.

Willoughby, C., Polatajko, H. and Wilson, B. (1995) The Self Esteem and Motor Performance of Young Learning Disabled Children. *Physical and Occupational Therapy in Pediatrics,* vol. 14, no. 3/4, 1–30.